Eat Out, Eat Right

*The Guide
to Healthier
Restaurant Eating*

THIRD EDITION

Hope S. Warshaw, MMSc, RD, CDE

Surrey Books
CHICAGO

Printed in Canada.

Library of Congress Cataloging-in-Publication Data

Warshaw, Hope S., 1954–

    Eat out, eat right : the guide to healthier restaurant eating /
Hope S. Warshaw. — 3rd ed.

        p.   cm.

    Summary: "Guide to healthy restaurant dining. Third edition
provides updated guidelines for making healthier menu choices
from a wide variety of foods and cuisines. Includes sample menus,
nutritional charts, and diabetic exchanges"—Provided by pub-
lisher.

    ISBN-13: 978-1-57284-092-8 (pbk.)

    ISBN-10: 1-57284-092-7 (pbk.)

    1. Nutrition. 2. Restaurants—United States. 3. Reducing diets.
I. Title.

RA784.W364 2008
613.2—dc22

                                        2007042185

10 9 8 7 6 5 4 3 2 1

Surrey is an imprint of Agate Publishing. Surrey books are available in bulk at
discount prices. For more information, go to agatepublishing.com.

Table of Contents

Dedication

To everyone who takes on the challenge of eating healthier restaurant meals and successfully implements the many skills and strategies in the pages ahead—may your efforts help you live a long and healthy life, and may our collective efforts lead to a wider array of healthier choices in restaurants and more options for smaller portions in the near future!

Acknowledgments

It should be no surprise that there are many people to thank in bringing the third edition of *Eat Out, Eat Right* to print.

Let me begin with a debt of gratitude and a big thanks to Susan Schwartz. Susan, who recently retired from publishing, was the owner of Surrey Books. Susan and I came together in 1988 because 20 years ago, she had the vision that healthy people and also those who are dealing with nutrition-related illnesses would benefit from detailed information about how to eat healthy in restaurants. Susan's desire to publish a book on the topic allowed me to publish my first book.

Another big thanks is in order for Doug Seibold. Doug is the owner of Surrey Books and Agate Publishing. Doug, a food lover who appreciates the value of nutritious and healthy eating, had the foresight to recognize that *Eat Out, Eat Right* is just what people, who are eating restaurant foods more than ever before, need to help them navigate the minefields of restaurant menus.

Thanks is also in order for Paula Payne, the registered dietitian who tirelessly helped me gather nutrition data from restaurants.

Last, but not least, is my near and dear family, Don and Hilary, who stood by me through the revision of this book—chapter by chapter—for months. Don't feel too sorry for them, though—they did get to enjoy eating out more often. I love you both!

Preface to 3rd Edition of
Eat Out, Eat Right

It has been nearly two decades since I began writing about and counseling people to make healthier choices when they eat restaurant foods. The response to *Eat Out, Eat Right* from consumers and health-care professionals has been gratifying. You have let me know that this practical and realistic advice is just what you need, as restaurant eating is often part of your daily food choices. It appears that you'll continue to need this advice, as the popularity of eating out will surely continue to grow in the years to come.

Although this book is small enough to carry around, it's full of helpful guidance. I've added even more tips and tactics to this 3rd edition, some of which I have personally tried and others that I have collected from readers and colleagues.

This 3rd edition of *Eat Out, Eat Right* integrates the many changes that have occurred in the constantly evolving restaurant industry. For example, a wider variety of foods are available as fast food. In addition to burgers and fries, you can now get pizza, Mexican, Chinese and even Middle Eastern food quickly. New chain restaurants open every day. More nutrition information is available from national and large regional restaurant chains via the Internet, which has allowed me to provide you with more snapshots of nutrition facts for most styles of restaurants.

As people have become more nutrition-conscious, some restaurants have aimed to offer healthier offerings. For instance, it's relatively easy to get lowfat milk and reduced-calorie or nonfat salad dressings at most restaurants. Special requests have become commonplace, and most establishments welcome you to split or share menu items in an effort to control portions or be creative with the menu.

Today, it's a bit easier to eat healthy in restaurants, but it's by no means simple. At most restaurants, the portion sizes continue to grow. Sometimes I, and I'm sure you do as well, feel like a fish swimming upstream as I try to eat healthy restaurant meals. However, if you put the 10 Skills and Strategies introduced on pages 27 to 35 to use and integrate all the tips and tactics in each chapter into your daily habits, you'll be on your way to healthier eating in restaurants in no time.

Good luck on your journey. My hope is that *Eat Out, Eat Right* makes eating healthy easier without diminishing the pleasure and enjoyment of restaurant dining. If we keep ordering healthier items and making special requests, restaurants will get the hint that the demand exists for healthy options and smaller portions. Speaking up and asking for what you want eventually can make a difference, so keep requesting the foods you want. Together, we'll create change.

Hope S. Warshaw, MMSc, RD, CDE
Author, *Eat Out, Eat Right*

Foreword

As Americans have become busier and more prosperous, the trend of eating out has become more popular than ever before. *Eat Out, Eat Right* is the third edition of an extraordinarily helpful guide to healthier restaurant eating. Why is this an important book? Because there is also a continuing trend among Americans to become more overweight, which also leads to such illnesses as type 2 diabetes, high blood pressure, heart disease, and strokes.

Although people tend to be somewhat more careful at home about what they eat, they often throw caution to the wind when they eat out. They choose large portions, high-calorie foods, sugary beverages, and rich desserts, which adds up to excess calories, saturated fat, cholesterol, and sugar.

This book does not discourage restaurant eating; in fact, it encourages it. *Eat Out, Eat Right* is a sane guide to navigating the waters of restaurant menus, including a diverse world of multicultural choices. Restaurants serving myriad ethnic cuisines are now everywhere, and they are worth exploring.

However, restaurant patrons should not be passive about where they go and what they order. There is nothing wrong with being selective. Restaurants that don't offer healthy options can easily be avoided. Set your own rules on what you will or won't eat. You can carefully select menu offerings, manage your portion sizes, and request that your food is prepared in a way that will retain its taste and the variety and ensure a healthier meal, but this requires some skill and some confidence. You can't go head-to-head with a server or chef unless you know what you want and what you are talking about.

Since Americans are eating out more and more, restaurant eating makes an impact on our health, but you can enjoy yourself, get your money's worth, and still eat healthy. Eating a 4-ounce steak instead of a 20-ounce one may not seem cost effective at the time, but making such choices can make it much easier to maintain your health. Overnutrition is a serious health problem in America: We ingest too many calories, too much cholesterol, too much fat, and too much sugar. It is a time for a change—a decrease in calories and an increase in physical activity.

Eat Out, Eat Right gives you the kind of knowledge you need to make practical, rational, and confident requests. It gives you the tools to order foods you like prepared the way you want them. You'll find the information you need about the foods restaurants offer, and how those foods are prepared. Hope Warshaw has written an excellent book that is practical, to the point, and easy to use, and I strongly recommend it. Rely on Hope Warshaw's book to help you savor the pleasure of dining out *and* improve your health.

Xavier Pi-Sunyer, M.D.
Professor of Medicine
St. Luke's-Roosevelt Hospital
Columbia University College of
  Physicians and Surgeons
New York, NY
September 2007

❖❖❖❖
❖

How to Use
Eat Out, Eat Right

The goal of *Eat Out, Eat Right* is to provide you with a straight-forward, easy-to-use, and realistic "hands-on" approach to making healthy choices when dining out. The tips, tactics, skills, and strategies presented in the pages ahead will help you select restaurants more carefully. Once you are in front of a menu board or have a menu in hand, you will be able to order healthier meals. This concise, to-the-point book is divided into three parts:

Part I is an overview. In it, you'll learn about how today's restaurant eating habits are changing our lives and health, and you'll discover why it's challenging to eat healthy restaurant meals—no matter what type of foods the restaurant offers. You'll gather skills and strategies to apply at all types of restaurants, whether they serve typical American fare or a fusion of ethnic cuisines. Part I also covers several other important topics, including: additional resources for nutrition information, making healthier beverage choices, and helping children develop healthier restaurant eating habits that will last them a lifetime.

Parts II and III have similarities. Part II contains the chapters that cover American style cuisine, including breakfasts at coffee shops or bakeries; lunches at fast-food joints, sandwich spots, or salad bars; and dinners at seafood restaurants or fine-dining establishments. Part III contains ethnic restaurants, including cuisines from Mexico, Italy, China, Thailand, Japan, India ... and more.

The chapters in Parts II and III are similarly organized to make the content easy to use. The elements below are provided for each chapter. Once you read a few chapters, you'll quickly learn how to zero in on the information you need.

- *The Menu Profile* is an overall description of the specific cuisine. You'll learn about its healthy assets and unhealthy liabilities. Also included is a selection—from soup to dessert—of what to order and what to avoid, as well as tips and tactics to get menu items prepared as you want—and need—them.
- *The Nutrition Snapshot* provides the nutrition facts for a sampler of the cuisine's typical dishes. Some of the mind-boggling numbers will shock you, but at the same time, the sampler will also help you realize that there are healthier choices. This data is culled from a variety of available sources; you can learn more about additional sources for restaurant nutrition information in Chapter 5.
- *Green flag words* are descriptors of healthier ingredients and cooking methods to look for when reading a menu. The more green flag words in a menu item's description, the better!
- *Red flag words* are descriptors of less healthy ingredients and cooking methods to look for when reading a menu. Carefully consider menu items with these words before ordering them.
- *Special Requests* are lists of specific phrases you can use to modify menu items so they are prepared exactly the way you want—and need—them.
- The *Typical Menu* is a cuisine-specific generic menu for

each type of food. *Typical Menus* lists commonly served offerings and checks off healthier choices.

♦ *May I Take Your Order* is a section in each chapter where you'll find two sample meals. One meal contains a lower-calorie option and the second contains a moderate-calorie option. These meals have been designed with the following daily healthy eating goals in mind:

– 50 percent of calories from carbohydrates
– 20 percent of calories from protein
– 30 percent of calories from fat
– No more than 300 milligrams (mg) of cholesterol
– No more than 3,000 milligrams (mg) of sodium

Low-calorie sample meals contain:

– 400–700 calories, based on a daily intake of 1,200–1,600 calories
– a cholesterol count of no more than 200 milligrams
– a sodium count of no more than 1,500 milligrams
– 30–35 percent fat calories

Moderate-calorie sample meals contain:

– 600–1,000 calories, based on a daily intake of 1,800–2,200 calories
– a cholesterol count of no more than 200 milligrams
– a sodium count of no more than 1,500 milligrams
– 30–35 percent fat calories

Each sample meal is also followed by a nutrition summary that provides a "guesstimate" of the meal's nutrient composition. This information is based on sample recipes, nutrient composition tables from the United States Department of Agriculture (USDA), and available nutrition information.

♦ *Menu Lingo* is specific to the restaurant cuisines in Part III, the ethnic restaurants. Menus in ethnic restaurants often have unfamiliar ingredient names, preparation styles, and menu items. Some chapters contain a glossary of menu terms. *Menu Lingo* helps you understand the cuisines and gives you more information to make healthier choices.

Eat Out, Eat Right is not a book to read cover to cover and then put on a shelf. It's a book you'll want to read through once and then keep close at hand when you eat out. Stash the book in your car's glove compartment, a desk drawer at work, your briefcase, or your purse.

1

Trends in Restaurant Eating and Foods

A Historical Glimpse

What a difference a few hundred years makes. In the taverns and boardinghouses of the 1700s, the focus was on serving alcohol, and food was often an afterthought. In the mid-1800s, full-service restaurants, such as Delmonico's in New York, began to open. Two hundred years ago, it was both a novelty and a rarity to sit down to dine on a hot meal outside of your home. Restaurant dining was primarily the reserve of wealthy individuals who lived in metropolitan areas.

In the mid-1900s, fast food was born, courtesy of Richard and Maurice McDonald. For many years after the McDonald's restaurant chain took off (and spawned many imitators), takeout orders other than fast-food meals were still unheard of, and people only dined out on special occasions. Restaurant meals were for celebrations: a birthday, an anniversary, or Mother's Day, when moms around the country were treated to a special meal.

Eating Out Today

Fast-forward another 50 years to today. According to the National Restaurant Association, Americans eat more meals out now than ever before—an average of 5 meals per week. Your count may be considerably higher. Restaurant meals are no longer enjoyed just in restaurants, and fast-food restaurants aren't the only options for to-go meals. Today, almost all restaurants offer meals to go, and many national chains designed as full-service restaurants also offer a special window or entrance for to-go orders.

According to a report requested and funded by the FDA from the Keystone Center entitled The Keystone Forum on Away-From-Home-Foods: Opportunities for Preventing Weight Gain and Obesity (http://www.keystone.org/spp/documents/Forum_ Report_FINAL_5-30-06.pdf), today Americans spend a greater percent of their food dollar away from home than ever before. National Restaurant Association statistics reveal that in 1970, 26 percent of every food dollar in America was spent in a restaurant. By 2006, the number had nearly doubled, to 48 percent. As a result, prepared food is much more readily available. Ready-to-eat meals are now available in restaurants, supermarkets, and even gas stations.

New Options for Dining

Restaurants help us get the job of eating done quickly and simply. That's why people flock to fast-food restaurants that now offer a wide range of fare, from burgers to Mexican cuisine, pizza and more. A new category of casual sit-down restaurants (which are called family-fare restaurants in *Eat Out, Eat Right)*, such as Chili's, Applebee's, and Ruby Tuesday, has grown exponentially. Sandwich shops offering subs, soups, and salads have also experienced explosive growth. At the same time, a wide mix of ethnic-food chains such as P.F. Chang's, Chipotle Mexican Grill, and Olive Garden, and independent restaurants now dot the landscape. These range from the well-entrenched ethnic favorites—Chinese, Mexican and Italian—to Japanese, Thai, and Middle Eastern, among others.

Coffee shops and bakery cafes appear on just about every street corner in metropolitan areas, and they dramatically expand the times of day that restaurants are crowded. They are usually bustling at mealtimes and nearly as busy throughout the day, serving snacks and big, bigger, and biggest coffee drinks.

No matter what type of restaurant you're contemplating, you'll find advice for healthier eating at all these establishments in the pages ahead.

Restaurant Foods and Health

Could this omnipresent availability of food be a factor in the epidemics of obesity and chronic diseases that have overweight as their root cause, such as heart disease, high blood pressure, and type 2 diabetes? There's no question about it: The aforementioned Keystone Forum report to FDA confirms it. According to the National Institutes of Health (NIH), 66 percent of American adults—133 million people—are overweight. About half of the people in this group are 30 percent above their desired body weight, and thus classified as obese.

Children and adolescents are not immune. According to national health surveys, approximately 14 percent of children two to five years old, and 17 percent of adolescents 12 to 19 years old, are overweight or obese. That's a three- and four-fold increase since 1976, respectively. A study of children and adolescents showed that a higher intake of fast food resulted in a higher likelihood of overweight and increased insulin resistance, which is a precursor to prediabetes and type 2 diabetes.

The American Diabetes Association (ADA) (www.diabetes .org) estimates that more than 20 million Americans have type 2 diabetes, and more than 50 million have a condition called prediabetes that is closely linked to overweight (in many cases, losing weight can make the condition disappear). The American Heart Association (www.americanheart.org) estimates that nearly 80 million Americans have one or more forms of cardiovascular disease (CVD), including high blood pressure, heart disease, and stroke. Additionally, health experts believe that almost half of adult Americans are at risk for cardiovascular disease and/or type 2 diabetes because they are overweight or obese.

Too Many Calories, Too Few Nutrients

In 1977, nutrition surveys showed that Americans consumed just under 20 percent of their calories away from home. In a 1994–1996 food intake survey, Americans reported that they consumed 32 percent of their calories away from home. The average American in 2008 eats an even greater percentage of his or her calories away from home.

Beyond just eating out more frequently, Americans often equate value with volume; as a result, they often consume an excess of calories in restaurant meals. "Meal deals" at many burger chains easily top 1,500 calories, depending on the size or ingredients of the burger, whether or not French fries are included and how much is consumed, and whether the drink contains sugar and how much is consumed.

Only a handful of studies have observed the food composition of restaurant meals. They conclude that most adults and children eat more calories and unhealthy saturated fat than they should and too few servings of healthy foods, such as fruits, vegetables, and lowfat milk. Do these findings surprise you? Probably not. As a result, it is a challenge to pick and choose from restaurant menus and come up with healthy meals.

Healthful and Helpful Restaurant Trends

Although it's not easy to find—or, more accurately, create—a healthy restaurant meal, some of the trends are beginning to change. Over the last few decades, health consciousness has grown slowly. At points when interest in healthier eating has been high, restaurant menus include more healthy options, such as lighter burgers, salads, lowfat milk, nonfat salad dressing and smaller portions. Over the years, some of the changes have stuck and others, such as McDonald's McLean burger and Taco Bell's Border Lights menu, have flopped because people simply didn't order the items.

Today, there is a renewed interest in healthy eating, and restaurants—especially national chains—are feeling the pressure to respond. Fast-food eateries now offer raw vegetables, yogurt, and fresh fruit as options in kids' meals. Attention is being paid to reigning in the extreme portion sizes available at so many restaurants: Consider T.G.I. Friday's "Right Size, Right Price" portion-controlled menu and McDonald's abandonment of the "Supersize" promotions that encouraged consumers to dramatically increase their meals' portion size for a marginal increase in cost.

Speaking of McDonald's, the chain is leading the charge toward healthy dining among fast-food establishments. McDonald's now offers an expanded list of healthier choices, including a variety of salads and wrap-style sandwiches for adults and kids' meal options like sliced apples with a lowfat dipping sauce, juice boxes, and carrot sticks.

Healthier drinks, such as bottled water, water, light lemonade and diet noncarbonated beverages, are now available in more restaurants. Starbucks Coffee has made it company policy to always use lowfat (2 percent) milk in its beverages unless a customer requests whole milk. On the whole, more restaurateurs are more open to honoring reasonable special requests to help you create healthier meals.

If you're interested in choosing healthier restaurant meals, you've picked up the right book. In the pages ahead, you'll learn key skills and strategies to eat healthfully in nearly any restaurant. But before you read on, take a few minutes to get to know your restaurant eating habits.

Get to Know Yourself

First, you must raise your awareness about how often you eat restaurant meals, what types of restaurants you choose, and what foods you choose at the restaurants you frequent. In Chapter 4, one of the strategies for healthy restaurant eating is *"Assess the whens, whys, wheres, and whats of your restaurant meals."* Being aware of your behaviors is the first step to changing behaviors. Think about your answers. What have you observed? Where do you need to start making changes? Choose a few easy changes first. Then, make a few more changes. Every so often, you'll want to come back to these questions about your restaurant eating habits. Observe your successes and think about what you want to change next. Remember, slow and steady changes can last a lifetime and help you achieve your health goals.

♦ What meals and snacks do you eat away from home, and how often do you eat out during the course of a day, week, or month? Consider weekdays and weekends and estimate the total number of prepared meals and snacks that you purchase. Don't forget meals and snacks that you purchase at restaurants and eat somewhere else.

_____

_____

_____

_____

_____

◆ Why do you eat restaurant meals? (Circle all that apply.)
  – Restaurant meals are convenient.
  – I don't like to cook.
  – I don't have/make time to cook.
  – I want to have someone serve me.
  – I enjoy a wide spectrum of ethnic flavors that I cannot create in my kitchen.
  – I need a place and way to get together with friends, family, or business associates.
  – I want to relax during lunch or at dinner after a long day.
  – I don't make time to make breakfast at home.
  – I don't make time to make my lunch at home and bring it to work.

◆ How many times a day, a week, or a month do you eat at or buy take-out at the types of restaurants listed below?
  – Fast food hamburger, chicken, or seafood chains _____
  – Pizza _____
  – Sandwich shops _____
  – Coffee shops _____
  – Family-fare _____
  – Steak house _____
  – Fine dining _____
  – Ethnic fare (fast food) _____
  – Ethnic fare (table service) _____
  – Sweets/desserts/ice cream _____

◆ What foods do you eat in the restaurants listed above, and in what amounts?

Record what you usually order in restaurants you frequent (and don't forget the beverages you drink).

_____

_____

_____

_____

_____

_____

_____

_____

_____

_____

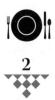

2

Take Healthy Eating Guidelines Out to Eat

Restaurant meals often invert healthy eating guidelines: They can be heavy in meat (protein), fats (total fat, saturated and *trans* fats), refined carbohydrates (including both nonwhole-grain starches and added sugars), and sodium. They're often lacking in whole grains, vegetables, lowfat dairy items, and fruit. In fact, the last two food groups are often nowhere to be found.

Consider the two meal comparisons below comparing one not-so-healthy and one healthier meal from two national chain restaurants. (The nutrition information used here is provided by the restaurants.)

Panera Bread

Not-so-healthy meal

Food / Amounts	Calories	Carbohydrate (g)	Protein (g)	Total Fat (g)	Saturated Fat (g)	*Trans* Fat (g)	Sodium (mg)
Cream of Chicken and Wild Rice Soup, 8 oz	200	19	5	12	8	0	970
Bacon Turkey Bravo Sandwich 1 whole	750	83	47	26	8	0	2720
Totals	950	102	52	38	14	0	3690

Healthier meal

Food / Amounts	Calories	Carbohy-drate (g)	Protein (g)	Total Fat (g)	Saturated Fat (g)	*Trans* Fat (g)	Sodium (mg)
Smoked Turkey Breast Sandwich, ½	230	24	15	8	1.5	0	840
Greek Salad, ½ portion	260	7	5	24	5.0	0	760
Fresh Fruit Cup, Small (5 oz)	70	19	1	0	0	0	15
Totals	560	50	21	32	6.5	0	1615

Panda Express

Less-Healthy Meal

Food / Amounts	Calories	Carbohy-drate (g)	Protein (g)	Total Fat (g)	Saturated Fat (g)	*Trans* Fat (g)	Sodium (mg)
Chicken Egg Roll, 1	170	17	8	8	1.5	0	410
Sweet and Sour Pork 5.5 oz/1 serving	400	35	13	23	4.5	0	360
Eggplant and Tofu in Garlic Sauce, 5.5 oz/1 serving	180	20	5	10	1.5	0	690
Fried Rice, 1 serving/8 oz	450	67	13	14	3.0	0	710
Totals	1200	139	39	55	11	0	2170

Healthier meal

Food / Amounts	Calories	Carbohydrate (g)	Protein (g)	Total Fat (g)	Saturated Fat (g)	*Trans* Fat (g)	Sodium (mg)
Veggie Spring Roll, 1	80	11	2	4	1.0	0	270
String Bean Chicken Breast 5.5 oz/1 serving	160	10	12	8	1.5	0	550
Broccoli Beef 5.5 oz/1 serving	150	11	11	7	1.5	0	510
Steamed White Rice ½ serving/4 oz	190	40	5	2	0	0	15
Totals	580	72	30	21	4	0	1345

Key Information

These two meal comparisons illustrate how restaurant meals can quickly become less than healthy with large portions, unhealthy food choices and high-fat ingredients. Observe how the following changes on the Panera Bread meal cut the calories, carbohydrates, saturated fat, and sodium by about half.

● Choosing a half sandwich with fewer high-fat ingredients instead of a whole sandwich with bacon, cheese, and a mayonnaise-based sauce.
● Opting for a salad instead of a cream-based soup.
● Taking advantage of a fresh-fruit salad.

Observe how the following changes to the Panda Express meal cut the calories, carbohydrates, and total and saturated fat by about half. Sodium remains high, but it has decreased by a third.

- Choosing a small vegetarian appetizer.
- Selecting lower-fat steamed rice and eating half portions.
- Choosing lower-fat entrées that offer more vegetables.

Nine Healthy Eating How-Tos

The latest iteration of the Dietary Guidelines for Americans (www.healthierus.gov/dietaryguidelines) were published by the government in 2005, and they were probably not earth-shattering to you. They are based on current research and knowledge about nutrition and physical activity, and also reflect a growing concern about overweight and physical inactivity among adults and children. These dietary guidelines mirror the nutrition recommendations from well-respected health associations including the American Heart Association, the American Cancer Society, and the American Diabetes Association.

But it is a challenge to make these straightforward, simplistic nutrition guidelines a part of your busy daily life. The fact that unhealthy foods are readily and quickly available and cheap only complicates matters. Below, you'll find the nine key healthy eating goals from the Dietary Guidelines for Americans. To the right of each goal, you'll find a few ways to put that guideline into practice in restaurants. Keep in mind that making small changes in your restaurant food choices and lifestyle can add up to big differences in the calories you consume and your long-term health outcomes.

#	Dietary Guideline and Interpretation	Tips to Implement Dietary Goals in Restaurants
1.	*Guideline:* Eat a variety of foods from the basic food groups and stay within your calorie needs. *Interpretation:* The basic food groups are considered to be whole grains, fruits, vegetables, lowfat dairy, meats, and fats. Ensure that most of the foods you eat are from these groups, and select a variety of foods within each basic food group. The foods in these groups are dense in nutrients; they pack in lots of vitamins and minerals.	• Get out of your comfort zone. There is a huge variety of foods available in restaurants, so test your palate with unfamiliar basic foods, such as roasted beets, bean and barley soup, or stone-ground whole-grain bread. • Seek out whole grains, vegetables, and fruits at restaurants. Next, look for preparations that reduce the fat content and added sugar count of these foods.
2.	*Guideline:* Control the amount of calories you eat to get to or stay at a healthy body weight. *Interpretation:* Don't eat more calories than your body needs each day. If you aren't at a healthy body weight now, trim your calories by eating less and increase the number of calories you burn. A healthy body weight is an important factor in your long-term health and for prevention of chronic diseases. Losing 5 to 10 percent of your current body weight can help you reduce many health risk factors.	• Portion control is king when you want to control restaurant calories. Split and share to your heart's content, order half portions, or take half of your meal home. • Be on the lookout for ways that fats creep into your restaurant foods. Fats are concentrated forms of calories and send the calorie count up.

#	Dietary Guideline and Interpretation	Tips to Implement Dietary Goals in Restaurants
3.	*Guideline:* Increase the amount of fruits, vegetables, whole grains, and nonfat or lowfat milk and milk products you eat each day. *Interpretation:* The foods that pack the greatest amount of vitamin and mineral punch are fruits, vegetables, whole grains, and lowfat dairy foods. However, these are the very foods Americans don't eat enough of. One reason: Restaurants generally have little to offer in these food groups.	• As fruit is often hard to find at restaurants, get the fruit you need elsewhere. Take a serving or two of fresh or dried fruit with you each day and consume it between or after meals. • If you plan to purchase a take-out or fast-food meal, bring along individually wrapped bags or portions of easy-to-carry vegetables, such as baby carrots, pre-cut carrots, cherry tomatoes, and celery sticks, or fruits, such as grapes or apples. • Opt for entrée salads as a main course or choose a side salad instead of chips or French fries. • Drink lowfat milk instead of soda or other calorie-laden beverages. • Include yogurt as a snack.
4.	*Guideline:* Choose fats wisely for good health. *Interpretation:* Today there is less focus on eating less fat (less than 30 percent of your calories) and more focus on choosing healthier fats. You can eat about 25 to 35 percent of your calories as fat as long as most of it is polyunsaturated or monounsaturated fats. Reduce the amount of saturated and *trans* fats (read more about *trans* fats below) you consume. Unfortunately, this is easier said than done with restaurant foods.	• Ask or observe what oil(s) are used at the restaurant. An increasing number of restaurants are now divulging this information. Liquid oils, such as soybean, corn, and canola oils, are commonly used. They are low in saturated fat and have no *trans* fats. • Avoid fried foods because they have high total fat content and a potential for *trans* fats (this is slowly changing as the type of oil used for frying changes). • Dip bread in tiny amounts of olive oil instead of using butter. • Always order salad dressing on the side and use very little of it. Olive oil and vinegar is a delicious dressing that is low in saturated fat and sodium. • Order items with lowfat preparations—grilled, barbecued, roasted, steamed, or poached.

#	Dietary Guideline and Interpretation	Tips to Implement Dietary Goals in Restaurants
5.	*Guideline*: Choose carbohydrates wisely for good health. *Interpretation*: Sources of carbohydrates range from unhealthy added sugars and refined carbohydrates to healthy whole grains. Americans eat about the right percent of calories from carbohydrate, but not the right kinds: too much added sugars and refined carbohydrates, and not enough whole-grain and high-fiber carbohydrates.	• Select whole-grain hot or cold cereals for breakfast. • Choose whole-grain breads or rolls for sandwiches. • Select a whole-grain roll from the bread basket. • Choose brown rice instead of white rice (when it's an option). • Enjoy a cup or bowl of bean soup or chili with beans. • Look for fresh fruit, fruit canned in its own juice, or 100 percent fruit juice. • Share desserts among many diners. • Choose low-calorie, sugar-free beverages. Water is a great healthy option. Diet beverages, black coffee, and unsweetened tea also have no calories or added sugar. Sweetened iced tea and coffee is an acceptable option as long as it is sweetened with a sugar substitute and/or lowfat milk.
6.	*Guideline*: Choose and prepare foods with little salt. *Interpretation*: Your sodium count should be no more than 2,300 milligrams per day. To accomplish this, eat fewer processed and prepared foods, which contribute about three quarters of all the sodium Americans eat. Do not add salt at the table.	• Don't salt your food at the table. • Beware of ingredients and sauces that load on the sodium: mayonnaise-based sauces, bacon, olives, cheese, pickles, and salad dressings. • When possible, choose fresh over processed foods. • Soups are high in sodium. • Fast foods are generally high in sodium. • Turkey breast and roast beef are lower in sodium than ham, salami, bologna and other sandwich meats and cold cuts.

#	Dietary Guideline and Interpretation	Tips to Implement Dietary Goals in Restaurants
7.	*Guideline:* If you drink alcoholic beverages, do so in moderation. *Interpretation:* Be moderate when it comes to alcohol—the calories add up fast. For women, this means no more than one drink per day and for men, no more than two drinks per day.	• You can moderate your alcohol intake by only drinking when you dine out. • Choose beer, wine, or a simple mixed drink rather than high-calorie mixed drinks with many ingredients. • Always have a noncaloric beverage, such as water, on hand so you can slowly sip your alcoholic drink. • Read more about managing alcoholic beverages in Chapter 8.
8.	*Guideline:* Keep food safe to eat. *Interpretation:* This guideline was included because the incidence of foodborne illnesses is on the upswing.	• Wash your hands before every meal. • Watch how the restaurant's workers handle foods when foods are made in front of you. Make sure they wear gloves and their hair is away from their faces. • If anything doesn't look or taste right, don't eat it. Send it back or throw it out. • Order wisely. Limit mayonnaise-based foods. Order foods that the restaurant is likely to use a lot versus a little.
9.	*Guideline:* Be physically active everyday. *Interpretation:* The connection between overeating and underexercising is clear. Adults are encouraged to be physically active at least 30 minutes a day, and children should be active for 60 minutes. Get a few minutes of activity here and there to reach your daily goals.	• Don't look for the closest parking space. Park as far as possible from the restaurant. • If you can walk to the restaurant, do so. • Take a stroll after an evening restaurant meal to burn off excess calories. • Get some extra exercise before you splurge.

More About Fats

Fat is a villain in restaurant foods from both a calorie and health standpoint, so it's important to understand the health goals regarding fats in more depth. As noted above, Americans are encouraged to eat between 25 to 35 percent of their daily calories as fat. For example, a person who eats about 1,500 calories per day should consume between 42 and 58 grams of fat. Most of these fat calories should come from polyunsaturated and monounsaturated fats, rather than saturated or *trans* fats. Polyunsaturated and monounsaturated fats are prevalent in liquid oils, such as olive, canola, corn, safflower, and soybean oils. They are also naturally found in some foods, such as nuts, meat, poultry, seafood, and dairy foods. Keep in mind that all foods that contain fat have varying amounts of healthy and less-healthy forms of fat. For example, although canola oil is a healthier oil to consume because of its high amount of poly- and monounsaturated fat, it also contains a small amount of saturated fat.

Saturated and *trans* fats have been shown to have an effect on blood lipids and cardiovascular disease. Foods that contain significant amounts of saturated fat are mainly derived from animal sources: cheese, red meats, poultry, seafood, whole milk, ice cream, and butter, for example. A few nonanimal-based oils, such as coconut, palm, and palm kernel oil, also contain significant amounts of saturated fats. These oils are often used in the production of crackers, cookies, baked goods, and fried snack foods.

Much attention has been paid to *trans* fat over the last few years because of its connection to cardiovascular disease. As a result, information about the level of *trans* fat in foods has been added to the government-mandated Nutrition Facts panel on most packaged foods. This attention to *trans* fat has encouraged some restaurant chains to provide the *trans* fat content of their menu offerings. The reality is that most Americans consume a fairly small amount of *trans* fat, but even that small amount is hazardous to the heart and blood vessels. About 80 percent of the *trans* fats Americans eat are from processed foods that contain partially hydrogenated vegetable oils, and only about 20 percent are occur naturally in animal-based foods, such as meats and dairy foods.

Restaurants are being pressured to rid their menus of *trans* fats altogether, and in some cities, *trans* fats have been banned from use by restaurants. Many fast-food chains have or are in the process of eliminating *trans* fats from their menus—but doing so is easier said than done. Suppliers of healthier oils are having a hard time keeping up with demand; healthier oils are often more expensive; and some of the oils that contain *trans* fats have a longer fry life, which means that they can be used longer before being changed out for fresh oil and are therefore more economical for the restaurants.

The current recommendation from many health authorities, including the Dietary Guidelines for Americans and the American Heart Association, is to eat no *trans* fats at all. The best way to do this is to avoid foods that contain the ingredient "partially-hydrogenated fat" as an ingredient. This also means limiting the use of margarine. If you have a choice between margarine, butter, or oil, use a liquid vegetable- or nut-based oil. Also, minimize the amount of fried restaurant foods as much as possible. Although restaurants are slowly moving to frying in *trans* fat-free oils, most shortenings still contain *trans* fats. An added plus to cutting out fried foods is that you'll also reduce your total fat and calories.

Calories and Servings of Foods You Need

How many calories do you need to eat each day? That's a challenging question to answer simply because people come in different sizes and burn different amounts of calories. There's no one right amount of calories for all adults or children. Generally, most adults need between 1,600 to 2,200 calories a day. However, this can range greatly depending on the following factors:

♦ age
♦ height
♦ current weight, and whether you want to lose weight or are at a healthy weight
♦ daily activity level
♦ type and amount of physical activity

The following provides the number of servings per day needed from the basic food groups at both the 1,600 and 2,200 calorie level, according to the Dietary Guidelines for Americans.

Basic Food Group	1,600 Calories	2,200 Calories
Fruits	1½ cups	2 cups
Vegetables	2 cups	3 cups
Grains (half of the grains per day should be whole grains)	5 ounce equivalents (Ex: 1 slice of bread = 1 ounce)	7 ounce equivalents
Lean meats and beans	5 ounces	6 ounces
Milk and yogurt	3 cups	3 cups
Oils (this includes oils added to foods during processing, cooking, or at the table)	22 grams or about 4 teaspoons	29 grams or about 6 teaspoons
Discretionary calories (represents calories from solid fats and added sugars)	132	290

As you change your restaurant eating habits, keep these healthy eating basics in mind. When you look at a menu, consider these questions:

- How can I get more vegetables at this meal?
- Can I ask for olive oil instead of butter or margarine to dip my bread in, or better yet, use no fats on the bread at all?
- Are whole-grain breads available?
- Can I reduce the total fat of my meal by leaving off an ingredient or two?
- Can I save half the meat of this meal for tomorrow's lunch because the serving is about twice as much as I should eat?
- Is there an appetizer, salad, or cup of soup that is healthy and will help fill me up and reduce the amount of entrée I eat?
- And many more...

You'll learn many more tips and tactics to eat healthier and be creative with restaurant menus as you read this book.

3

The Pitfalls of Healthier Eating Out

Whether you're dining for pleasure on upscale cuisine that mixes ingredients and flavors from many cultures, blending business with lunch at a sit-down restaurant that serves traditional American fare, or grabbing a quick lunch or dinner from a fast-food restaurant or food court, the 10 pitfalls of healthier restaurant eating are common to all restaurant meals.

As you become aware of these 10 pitfalls, you'll learn that although they present challenges, they aren't insurmountable. The 10 skills and strategies provided in Chapter 4 will help you avoid them. As you read the rest of *Eat Out, Eat Right,* you'll learn more about specific pitfalls that you will encounter at each particular type of cuisine or style of restaurant. Gradually, you'll arm yourself with explicit skills and strategies to meet these challenges head on.

The 10 Pitfalls of Restaurant Foods

1. *Treating every restaurant meal as a special occasion.* A few decades ago, restaurant meals were reserved for special occasions. Other than these special occasions, meals were usually eaten at home. Today, people eat restaurant meals an average of five times a week. With this increased frequency of restaurant meals, you can't afford—weight-wise or health-wise—to order with a special-occasion mindset. You can still enjoy splurging

on occasional celebrations, but to keep your waistline from expanding and stay healthy, you'll have to tow the calorie line and integrate the healthy-eating basics covered in Chapter 2.

2. *Limited access to the chef.* In fine-dining restaurants, most of the food preparation is done from scratch—meaning starting with basic ingredients. As the meal is prepared, sauces and seasonings are added. In order to make changes to the specific way that the meal is prepared, you must have a willing chef. In some fast-food restaurants, the food arrives from the distributor almost completely prepared. In these situations, you have less control, but you can still exert pressure to get foods your way. Control these varied dining situations by asking questions and requesting changes. Restaurants need and want your business, and today they are more open than ever before to meet your needs. So get ready to speak up.

3. *Fruits, vegetables, whole grains, and lowfat dairy options can be hard to find.* The very foods we should be eating more of are often hard to find at restaurants. This includes fruits, vegetables, whole grains and lowfat dairy foods.

- You can now find salads in most fast-food restaurants, and side and entrée salads are usually well represented on menus at family-fare restaurants. In fine-dining establishments, however, vegetables are often only small side dishes, so you'll have to work to satisfy your requirement of two cups of vegetables per day.
- The only fruit in some restaurants is camouflaged between two crusts, so you'll need to eat fruit with meals you eat at home, or bring it with you to enjoy during the day.
- Whole grains are beginning to appear on menus of sandwich shops and better restaurants. You'll see whole-

wheat or grain breads available at most sub and sandwich shops. You may find whole grain choices in a basket of dinner rolls at better restaurants, but they are harder to find in ethnic restaurants.

• Lowfat dairy foods, such as milk or yogurt, can be challenging to find. Today, most fast-food restaurants and family-fare restaurants offer lowfat milk, which is better than whole milk, but few offer nonfat or skim milk. Milk is still fairly rare at ethnic restaurants. Yogurt—particularly healthier and lower-sugar plain yogurt—is not found in restaurants very often, but you'll find it served with Middle Eastern fare often. Lowfat milk and lower-fat and lower-sugar yogurts are available in individual servings at supermarkets and convenience stores, so you can make an extra stop to combine them with a take-out meal or integrate them as snacks between meals.

4. *Meats take center stage.* Meat often dominates the plate, particularly when it comes to American cuisine. (Meat is used as a general term in this book to include beef, lamb, pork, veal, poultry, and seafood.) As most people decide what they will order, they first consider the entrée, which will take center stage on the plate. Invariably, that means the meat. Healthy eating guidelines suggest that the meat portion per meal should be no more than 3 ounces (cooked) for most adults. Unless you order an appetizer or mixed dish with vegetables and starches (such as a stir-fry dish with noodles or a pasta dish), you'll get served a portion that is closer to 6 to 10 ounces.

Some cuisines, such as Asian or Mexican, often use smaller portions of meat. In most family-fare restaurants, you should share your meal, request a take-home container, or order appetizers to avoid large portions of meat. Meat should move from center stage to a supporting role: It should take up about a quarter of the plate, with half containing vegetables and the other quarter containing a healthy starch.

5. *Portions are way too big.* It seems that the "value equals volume" concept is here to stay in America. Portions, and the plates to hold them, just keep getting bigger. When you are served large portions, it's often difficult to stop eating when there's still food on your plate. A strategy to outwit large portions you'll read over and over in this book is to *control the portions when you order.* If less food is sitting in front of you, you will eat less food. Reducing your portion size should be your primary goal.

6. *Fats and oils are in, on, around, and through the meals you are served.* Fats and oils make foods taste good and stay moist. That's why such a wide variety of oils, fats, and other high-fat ingredients are used in restaurant foods from the start of the meal to the finish. You may start a meal in a family-fare restaurant with bread and butter or olive oil. In a Mexican restaurant, it may be chips and salsa. In a Chinese restaurant, it might be fried Chinese noodles. The butter, chips, and noodles all contain a lot of fat—which means a hefty bunch of calories.

In the kitchen, chefs use oil or butter to cook vegetable, grain, and starch dishes. Some even soak meat in pads of butter and herbs on the grill. Burgers and sandwiches are often partnered with high-fat ingredients, such as cheese or bacon. On top of that, a special sauce may be added, which usually starts with mayonnaise and finishes with many extra calories. A heavy pour of salad dressing can negate all the benefits of a salad's healthy fresh vegetables. Sour cream and butter get dumped on baked potatoes, and cream sauces drown meats and pastas. Food gets fried, stuffed, and smothered—typically with high-fat ingredients that pack on the calories. Controlling the amount of fat in your restaurant foods is key to healthier restaurant eating.

7. *Unhealthy fats and oils abound.* Of course, it is important to not eat too much total fat, but it's also important to eat more of the right types of fat—poly- and mono-unsaturated fat—and less of the wrong types of fat—saturated fat and *trans* fat. Many restaurants fry foods in oils that contain processed *trans* fats, but this is beginning to change as awareness grows about the dangers of *trans* fats. (Read more about *trans* fats and how to limit them in Chapter 2.)

Although it is not the same thing as fat, cholesterol in the foods you eat is another factor to consider. Limiting cholesterol from foods helps keep your total blood cholesterol and LDL (bad) cholesterol levels down. Cholesterol is only found in animal-based foods, such as dairy foods, egg-based foods, and meats of all kinds, including seafood. Keeping your portions of these foods small and enjoying some of them only occasionally helps reduce your cholesterol intake.

8. *Sodium levels often top the charts.* The Dietary Guidelines recommend only 2,300 milligrams of sodium per day. A quick check of the average restaurant meal's sodium level shows why people are consuming far too much sodium. Excess amounts of sodium are used primarily for two reasons: because it makes foods taste good, and because it is also an excellent preservative that extends the shelf life of foods.

Here's a few tricks to control the amount of sodium you eat at restaurants: Limit foods that are high in sodium, such as soup, cold cuts, fast-food chicken products, and French fries; high-sodium ingredients, such as anchovies, olives, and pickles; and high-sodium toppers, such as salad dressing, cheese sauces, or mayonnaise-based sauces. Don't use the salt shaker. And don't forget: If you eat less, you'll consume less sodium *as well as* fewer calories.

9. *Nonalcoholic beverages are big, bigger, and biggest.* Usually, the nonalcoholic beverages available in most fast-food and family-fare restaurants are sweetened (usually with high-fructose corn syrup) drinks, such as soda, lemonade, iced tea, and fruit-flavored drinks. The portions come in three sizes: big, bigger, and biggest. These sugary drinks add a large amount of undesirable added sugars and hundreds of calories with no nutrition value. Additionally, the incredible popularity of coffee beverages both hot and cold have dramatically added to Americans' intake of added sugars and unhealthy fats (including whole milk, half-and-half, and whipped cream). Healthier nonalcoholic beverage options are explored in Chapter 7.

10. *Alcoholic beverages run up calories and run down your resistance.* Alcohol seems to go hand-in-hand with sit-down and fine dining. At a business or celebration dinner, a person might enjoy a cocktail, a beer or a glass of wine, and perhaps an after-dinner drink. The result is hundreds of excess calories with no nutritional value. For some, consuming alcohol also weakens their resolve to eat healthfully. Learn ways to minimize the alcoholic-beverage calories you consume in Chapter 8.

Continue on to Chapter 4 to master skills and strategies to combat these 10 pitfalls.

4

Skills and Strategies for Healthier Eating Out

At this point, you may believe that the phrase "a healthy restaurant meal" is an oxymoron. After reading about the 10 pitfalls of restaurant meals, maybe you threw up your hands and thought that eating healthy restaurant meals is next to impossible. But that's not true at all!

If you have the will, and the skills and strategies you'll master in the pages ahead, *you can choose* to eat healthier restaurant meals. *You can choose* are the operative words in that sentence. As you put these skills and strategies for healthier eating out into practice day after day and begin to experience some of the health benefits, your job will get easier.

These 10 skills and strategies can be applied to just about any restaurant eating situation—whether you are eating in or taking out. These skills and strategies range from the psychological—changing your mindset about restaurant meals—to the practical—when and how to put your knife and fork down and push yourself away from the table.

1. *Develop a healthy mindset and a can-do attitude.* Developing a healthy mindset and being positive about eating healthier restaurant meals is the first critical step. Until you accomplish this step, you'll have a difficult time putting the other nine skills and strategies into action.

- Do you approach every restaurant meal as a special occasion?
- Do you cast caution and care to the wind, choose whatever your taste buds desire, and eat until you are stuffed?
- Do you use frequent restaurant meals as opportunities to reward yourself—and invariably partake in a fat-drenched appetizer or a decadent dessert?
- Do you think that you might as well get your money's worth and eat all that is on your plate?

After you've considered and honestly owned up to your present attitudes, think about the steps you can take to develop a healthier mindset about restaurant meals. Ask yourself what changes will help you find a balance between continuing to enjoy restaurant dining and ordering and eating healthier foods. Be kind to yourself: These changes will take some time and a lot of positive experiences.

2. *Assess the whens, whys, wheres, and whats of your restaurant meals.* Get to know your restaurant eating habits. Raising your awareness about your behaviors is the first step to changing them. Review the questions under the section "Get to Know Yourself" on page X of Chapter 1.

3. *Select a restaurant with care.* Choose restaurants that make it easier for you to eat healthfully. The reality is that you can choose to eat healthfully in almost all restaurants, but some menus make it easier than others. Steer clear of favorite restaurants where you usually eat unhealthy meals and healthy choices are rare, such as a fried-chicken or fish-and-chips restaurant.

4. *Think through your action plan.* "Think before you act" should be your *modus operandi*. If you are familiar with the menu offerings at a particular restaurant, preplan your order before you cross the restaurant's threshold. Be the first in your

party to order, which reduces the risk that you will make changes to your order as you listen to the orders of your dining companions. If you want to split or share menu items, say so as your fellow diners peruse their menus. Usually, others will be pleased you made the offer.

Also think about your menu choices in the context of your day. Ask yourself:

- ◆ "Have I eaten enough servings of fruits and vegetables?"
- ◆ "Will I be eating more meat at another meal?"
- ◆ "How much fat will I eat today?"

A preplanning concept that might help is calorie or nutrient banking, which you can use to monitor your intake of any dietary measure—calories, fats, carbohydrates, fruits, and vegetables. Calorie and nutrient banking teaches you to think about your food intake more than one meal at a time—and, if necessary, more than one day at a time. For example, if you plan to celebrate your anniversary at a swanky restaurant, you can "save" fat grams for days to "spend" on a special sauce or a favorite dessert.

One caution when using banking strategies: Don't fall into the trap of starving yourself prior to a restaurant meal. This practice is clearly a setup to overeat, and it usually backfires. For one thing, you will be extremely hungry, and you will weaken your resistance to unhealthy foods and extras.

Another way to bank calories is through increasing your physical activity. Increase your activity and burn more calories prior to or after meals by spending more time at the gym, taking long walks, swimming, or taking a nice after-dinner stroll.

5. *Be a "fat detector."* Dodging the fats in restaurants is a big challenge. Fat adds significant calories without adding any food

volume (or "bites"). A great example is a medium baked potato, which contains about 100 calories. Each teaspoon of regular butter or margarine contains 50 calories, and two tablespoons of regular sour cream adds 50 calories. Without adding a single bite, you can quickly add 150 calories to the baked potato.

Fat is the most saturated form of calories, at nine calories per gram. Carbohydrate and protein contain half the calories, with only four calories per gram. Therefore, even lowering fat intake by just a little can make a big impact on the number of calories you consume.

Learn to be a fat detector. Consider fats on the menu and on the table. "On-the-menu" fat appears in the ingredients used in cooking and food preparation—butter, oil, cream, sour cream, mayonnaise—and the foods themselves, like sausage on pizza, prime rib, and pork spareribs. Certain preparation methods, such as "deep-fried," "smothered," or "covered with a cream-based sauce," mean that the foods are drenched in fat. On ethnic menus, examples of words that mean "loaded with fat" include "Alfredo sauce" in an Italian restaurant, or "chimichangas," which are deep-fried burritos, in a Mexican restaurant. Become acquainted with high-fat items and learn which ingredients, preparation methods, and menu descriptions signal lowfat and healthy in each cuisine. (You'll find these in most of the chapters in Parts II and III.) Don't forget: Feel free to ask your server or order-taker questions about unfamiliar ingredients, preparations, and menu descriptions.

Fat creeps in "at the table" in several ways. When you sit down at a table, you may be greeted with rolls and butter, chips and salsa, Chinese noodles, or garlic bread. Even before you order, the fat begins to add up. Extra fats might also come in the form of sour cream, butter, margarine, mayonnaise, salad dressing, and added cream or milk in coffee. If all your dining companions agree, the best advice is to limit the fats at the table. Keep the rolls, but return the butter.

Your job as a fat detector becomes easy when you use *Eat Out, Eat Right.* In Parts II and III, the cuisine chapters include lists of "red flag" and "green flag" words. The red flag words are categorized by ingredients, preparation methods, and menu descriptions, and they indicate that dishes are high in fat and calories. Green flag words are also categorized by ingredients, preparation methods, and menu descriptions, and they indicate that dishes are lower in fat and calories.

6. *When you order, keep your healthy-eating goals in mind.* You were introduced to the nine keys to healthy eating in Chapter 2. Review these on occasion, and keep them in mind as you select restaurant meals. More than likely, you'll begin to integrate more fruits and vegetables and lighten up on your portions of meats and fats.

7. *Practice portion control from the get-go.* Large portions are a fact of life in restaurant dining. You'll need to "outsmart" the menu to cut portions down to a healthy size. A successful strategy is to control portions from the point of ordering. Think of this as the "out of sight, out of mouth" technique. It's a lot more difficult to control the amount you eat if food is just a forkful away. If it's not an option to reduce the portion size when you order, ask your server to bring you a take-home container when he or she brings the meal. You can divide the meal in half before you even begin to eat.

As you read *Eat Out, Eat Right,* you'll learn ways to control portions in specific types of restaurants. Your goal is to eat smaller quantities of the foods you enjoy. Here are a few general tactics:

- Steer clear of menu descriptions that indicate a large portion, such as jumbo, grande, supreme, extra large, king size, double, triple, feast, or combo.
- Go for the menu descriptions that indicate smaller servings, such as regular, petite, appetizer-size, kiddie, or queen-size.
- Ask for half, lunch, or appetizer portions.
- Choose from à la carte items and/or side offerings. Mix and match these to wind up with small servings of a few items.

8. *Get creative with the menu.* To eat healthful foods in reasonable portions, you'll need to be creative with menus. Get started with these few general creative tips, and in the cuisine chapters, you'll get more menu-specific ways to be creative.

- No rule says you must order an entrée. Mix and match items from the soups, salads, appetizers and side dishes on menus. There are countless ways to build meals with smaller portions.
- Order a cup of broth-based soup, like chicken with rice or bean and barley, or a side salad as a low-calorie filler, especially if your dining companions are enjoying high-fat appetizers.
- Opt for a side salad and an appetizer, and ask the server to serve your appetizer as the main course.
- Order two appetizers—one to eat as a first course and the other as your main course.
- Split portions with your dining companions. Feel free to order many courses—from soup to dessert—but split everything down the middle. In better restaurants, ask the server to split the items they can in the kitchen and serve them on separate plates.

- Eat "family-style." This is the primary eating style in many Asian restaurants, but it can be used in any restaurant. Order one or two fewer entrées than the total number of people who are dining.
- Share nutritionally complementary dishes. For example, in an Italian restaurant, one person could order Pasta Primavera, a vegetarian dish, and the other could order Chicken Marsala. The chicken dish would probably have at least 6 to 8 ounces of chicken, which is enough meat for two. The pasta dish would provide plenty of starch for two people and a healthy dose of vegetables as well.

9. *Order foods the way you want them.* If you want a dish prepared a special way, you must speak up and ask for it. A special request might mean asking that an ingredient, such as cheese, bacon, or sour cream, be deleted from the recipe. It may mean asking for a substitution, such as a baked potato instead of French fries or potato chips, or mustard instead of mayonnaise on a sandwich. Another wise special request is asking for an ingredient, like salad dressing, butter, or guacamole, to be served on the side, so you can control how much you eat. Perhaps your request is a cooking instruction, such as, "Please broil my fish with a small amount of butter," or "Use very little oil in my stir-fry." Assume that there's no harm in asking, and the worst someone can say is no.

You might think that you are ruffling feathers. However, there are ways to approach special requests that will put you at ease and won't embarrass you or your dining companions.

- Be reasonable and realistic. Don't try to completely remake a menu item by deleting several items and requesting several others.
- Request simple changes or additions. For instance,

request that salad dressing, sour cream, or a sauce be served on the side, or ask that French fries be replaced with a baked potato.

• Be pleasantly assertive. Let the server know what you want by using nonthreatening words. The following phrases can be very effective:
  – "Do you think the chef would ...?"
  – "I'd really appreciate it if you could ...?"
  – "May I have ... on the side?"
  – "Would it be a problem to substitute ... for ...?"

10. *Know when to say "enough."* You already know that portion control is the key to healthier restaurant meals. Control portions from the start by ordering creatively. If the portions are huge, request a take-home container and immediately set aside the portion to take home. If you feel uncomfortable doing so, separate the portion you don't want to eat and place it on a small plate, offer your dining companions "tastes," or just move the unwanted food to the side of your plate.

Be clear about your definition of fullness. Many people respond to external, rather than internal, cues. An external cue is food left on your plate. An internal cue is a full stomach. Learn to listen to your internal signals: How does your stomach feel when you have had enough to eat? Recognize this sensation as a message to put down your knife and fork instead of waiting for the unpleasant stuffed-turkey feeling. Slow the pace of your eating so your stomach has a chance to communicate to your brain that you are full. Last, take time to enjoy the taste of the food in your mouth. You don't need to be a member of the clean-plate club.

Enjoy the nonfood pleasantries of restaurant eating. If you focus exclusively on your food because of time constraints, hunger, or other stresses, you might miss enjoying the surrounding environment. Train yourself to enjoy all aspects of the restaurant experience, even if it's just a few minutes of relaxation or conversation with a friend. Think about all the upsides to dining out: no cooking, no packaging of leftovers, and no dirty dishes. Enjoying the nonfood pleasantries makes it easier to limit portions and eat healthfully.

5

Restaurant Nutrition Information— What's Available, and What's Not?

Thanks to the Internet and consumers' persistence, more nutrition information for restaurant foods is available than ever before. Although most regional and national chain "walk-up-and-order" restaurants provide detailed nutrition information, family-fare and other "sit-down-and-order" chains are less likely to provide this information. Independent restaurants—including everything from small ethnic take-out joints to fine-dining establishments—are even less likely to provide this information.

In this chapter, you will learn what nutrition information is available and how to access it. You will learn how to estimate how much food you are eating and see how activists are pushing the restaurant industry to make more nutrition information available.

What's Available at Walk-Up-and-Order Restaurants

You should be able to find detailed nutrition information for most walk-up-and-order national and large regional chain restaurants, which include conventional and ethnic fast-food restaurants, pizza joints, sub shops, and chicken chains. Most bagel and coffee shops also provide nutrition information for their foods.

You can reliably find most of this information on the restaurants' websites. Usually, it is easy to find: Most chain restaurant websites have a link on the home page like "Nutrition Information," "Nutritional Data," or a similar phrase. Some chains' websites even include meal calculators, which allow you to calculate nutrition totals for an entire meal. Some websites also allow you to add or subtract various ingredients to get totally customized calculations. Several national chains also place nutrition information posters on their walls or provide brochures with nutrition data. However, website nutrition information is usually more reliable because it is usually more up to date.

Most restaurants provide the following nutrition information: calories, grams of total fat, saturated fat, carbohydrates, cholesterol, sodium, and protein. Some chains also provide *trans* fat content.

What's Available at Sit-Down-and-Order Restaurants

Unfortunately, nutrition information for sit-down-and-order national restaurant chains is harder to find. If the chains serve healthier dishes, they will probably provide extensive nutrition data for those items—and little to no data about the rest of the menu. Several large sit-down chains do tell all, including P.F. Chang's, Denny's and Fazoli's. Ruby Tuesday provided nutrition information on tables during the low-carb craze, but the company has now removed it. You can find some nutrition information on the Ruby Tuesday website, but it is incomplete. The website for the Chili's chain has fairly detailed nutrition data, but it is challenging to find it (it is a small link on the restaurant's menu page).

No Numbers for Independent Restaurants

For the most part, nutrition data is not available for independently owned restaurants. Obtaining nutrition information properly is an expensive proposition and requires considerable effort, which is a compelling reason why only national chains make the effort.

Accessing Missing Info

There are a few other ways to gather the inside scoop on what you are eating. If you are particularly interested in getting nutrition data for a few menu items from a chain restaurant that doesn't publish its information, contact the chain's headquarters. They might be willing to provide you with answers for particular items.

Independent cafés, sandwich shops, and cafeterias use many packaged foods that feature the same Nutrition Facts panels found on the food products you buy. Ask your server if you can see the Nutrition Facts panels for foods you regularly eat.

More Info Online at Your Fingertips

The following websites offer an extensive amount of nutrition information for restaurants. Use these after you have made sure that the restaurant chains do not offer their own nutrition information.

◆ Calorie King (www.calorieking.com) offers the most extensive food and nutrition database around. You can purchase a downloadable version of the database for your PDA.

◆ Diet Facts (www.dietfacts.com) is a site dedicated to publishing nutrition data for people with diabetes and others who are interested in making healthy choices.

◆ Dottie's Weight Loss Zone (www.dwiz.com) includes information provided directly by restaurants and information obtained by consumers. Weight Watchers points are included for many items.

◆ Healthy Dining Finder (www.HealthyDiningFinder.com) allows you to search for restaurants that offer a selection of healthier menu items and view the nutrition information for those dishes. You can search by zip code and/or other criteria. The site was developed with a grant from the Centers for Disease Control and Prevention (CDC) and in collaboration with the National Restaurant Association. New restaurants are added regularly.

◆ NutritionData (www.nutritiondata.com) is provided by Condé Nast publications.

When No Facts Are Available, Make Educated Guesses

In the pages ahead, you'll find detailed nutrition information for many menu items. You'll also learn how to make educated guesses—guesstimates—about menu items for which there is no information. Here are a few tips to help you develop these skills.

◆ *Use measuring equipment at home.* Keep measuring cups and spoons and a food scale on your kitchen counter, where you're more likely to use them. Get in the habit of weighing and measuring your foods when you eat at home. Put the amount of pasta, rice, or potatoes you usually eat in a measuring cup to check how much you usually eat. Weigh your meat portions: Are they the correct size or too much? The more you familiarize yourself with the proper portion sizes, the better you'll be able to estimate restaurant food portions.

◆ *Use "handy" hand guides.* No matter where you are, you always have a guide—or two—to estimate portions. Parts of your hands can be used to estimate portion sizes of food. Take note that these guidelines serve as estimates. Think about these guidelines in relation to your own hands and then customize them, because usually, men have larger hands and women have smaller hands.

- The distance from the tip of the thumb to the first knuckle = 1 teaspoon
- The distance from the tip of the thumb to the second knuckle = 1 tablespoon
- The palm of the hand (width and thickness) = a cooked 3 ounce portion of meat. Objects that are of comparable size include a deck of cards, a bar of soap, or a computer mouse.
- A tight fist = ½ cup. A tennis ball is roughly the same size. Objects that are of comparable size to a ¼-cup (or 2 tablespoon) portion include golf and ping-pong balls.
- Loose fist or an open handful = 1 cup. Objects that are of comparable size include a baseball or softball.

♦ *Seek out nutrition information for similar foods.* If you are unable to estimate the nutrition information for restaurant foods you frequently eat, look for the Nutrition Facts labels for similar foods that are available in supermarkets, convenience stores, or restaurants that do provide nutrition information. This strategy can at least give you a ballpark estimate.

♦ *Unique challenges of ethnic foods.* It's especially hard to determine nutrition data for ethnic foods because so many ethnic restaurants are independently owned. Some nutrition information is available from a few of the large national ethnic eatery chains—P.F. Chang's for Chinese food, for example. Their numbers can help you guesstimate what your local favorite's numbers are. Other strategies are to look for similar frozen foods in your supermarket or review similar recipes in ethnic cookbooks, which may or may not include nutrition data but surely include ingredient lists. If you know what ingredients are used, you can make estimates.

Activists Push for Point of Purchase Nutrition Information

In 1994, the Nutrition Labeling and Education Act (NLEA) required detailed nutrition data to be provided by manufacturers of packaged foods, but little in this legislation encouraged restaurants to be more candid about the nutrition information for their foods. The only stipulation of the legislation that affects restaurants requires them to provide nutrition information to customers when nutrition and health claims are being used to market the foods. For example, if a restaurant describes a particular food as low-carbohydrate, lowfat, *trans* fat-free or even just "healthy," the nutrition information for the food must reflect the Food and Drug Administration's definition of the term, and the restaurant must be able to provide consumers with the nutrition information.

Activists, such as the food and nutrition watchdog group Center for Science in the Public Interest (www.cspinet.org), are fighting for legislation that forces all restaurant chains to provide nutrition information on the menu or menu board. Consider getting involved and being a change agent in your area.

6

Healthier Eating Out with Children

Children growing up today will probably eat restaurant meals more frequently than ever before. They're eating out more often for the same reasons that everyone is: their families have busy lives and 24/7 access to ready-to-eat foods.

Because children are eating in restaurants more frequently, they need to know how to plan healthy meals when they are out. Unfortunately, too many children today are already overweight or have increased risk of becoming overweight and developing related health disorders. Frequent restaurant meals have been proven to contribute to the risk of being or becoming overweight for all people, including children and adolescents. Several research studies have assessed how frequent restaurant meals impact the overall quality of the food that children and adolescents consume. This research has shown that when young people consume more restaurant food—often fast food—they eat more calories, total fat, and saturated fat. As you might guess, they get fewer servings of fruits, vegetables, and milk.

As a parent, grandparent, or other person involved in a child's life, you have an opportunity to teach healthy restaurant eating habits from the start. Don't give them a chance to learn unhealthy habits first. Show them how to select healthier menu items and put healthier eating skills and strategies into action. These habits will serve them well through their life.

Those Kids' Menus

Kids' menus invariably list kid-friendly and kid-favorite foods. Unfortunately, most of those kid-friendly foods are processed, loaded with fat, and overflowing with calories. If you are a parent, you could probably name the menu items in your sleep: the sandwiches include hamburgers, cheeseburgers, hot dogs, and grilled cheese. Each are usually served with either French fries or chips. Other entrées may include macaroni and cheese, pizza, pasta with tomato sauce, fried chicken fingers, or fried fish. They're almost always accompanied with a regularly sweetened carbonated soft drink. The only plus of kid's menus comes through in fast-food restaurants as the smaller portions … a benefit that can be shared by adults seeking smaller portions as well.

Where are the vegetables, whole grains, fruits, and cups of lowfat milk? They're nowhere to be found in most restaurants. Fortunately, some of the fast-food chains have begun to adopt healthier side items for kids' meals: They are trying to integrate fruits and vegetables into kid's meals in the form of baby carrots, apple slices, or applesauce.

Repeatedly offering children these supposed kid-favorite, less-healthy foods causes several problems. One, they quickly develop a taste for high-fat foods and don't eat as healthy as they should at home or away. Two, they don't get exposed to a wide array of foods. Eventually, there will be a very short list of foods that they will agree to eat. Let's widen, not narrow, the horizons of our kids' palates!

If you can limit the use of kids' menus, do so—especially in sit-down restaurants. As a family, develop some healthy restaurant eating guidelines, skills, and strategies, and make sure that every member of your family buys in to the idea. Think about using the following list as a starting point.

**Tips to Help Kids (and Their Families)
Eat Healthy in Restaurants**

♦ Make healthy eating in restaurants a family affair. If you eat out frequently (a couple of times a week or more), continue the healthy eating habits you practice at home when you are out in restaurants.

♦ Be a role model for your children. As the sayings go, "Monkey see, monkey do," and "Actions speak louder than words." If your children see you ordering healthy foods and not overeating, they will probably follow your lead. Be a constant and consistent role model. Over time, they acquire their own healthy eating habits.

♦ Limit the use of kids' menus unless they will help your children eat smaller portions or healthier foods, and/or fit in some healthier fruits and vegetables.

♦ Order from the main menu and eat family-style. Order fewer entrées than there are people at the table, and put the entrées in the middle of the table and request empty plates for everyone. Sharing the entrées is fun and allows children to explore more flavors.

♦ Help your kids eat smaller portions by encouraging them to choose from the soups, salads, appetizers, and side dishes. Mix and match for a healthy, palate-pleasing meal that's just the right size.

♦ Practice portion control when eating in fast-food restaurants or sandwich shops. When dining on fast-food burgers and fries, split a larger order (medium or large size) of fries between several or all family members. Order one sandwich and split it, and split the sides as well. That should be enough for you and one child.

♦ Divide up desserts. Kids love sweets, but they don't need a whole dessert to themselves. A few sweet bites for all family members are enough.

- Expose your children to a variety of foods and flavors. Widen the scope of foods they enjoy instead of limiting them to what adults believe are "kids' foods." Expand their palates with such delights as Mexican, Chinese, Italian, Thai, Middle Eastern, or Indian food. Sharing foods from around the world with your children helps them increase their perspective of the world and learn about different cultures.

- Develop some family guidelines for trying new foods, such as insisting that children try at least a few bites of everything. This guideline can apply at home and away.

- Encourage your children to choose nutrient-dense beverages or water. Most restaurants offer lowfat milk. Make milk the first choice if you are at home or out, because kids need milk for calcium, Vitamin D, and other essential nutrients. Fruit juice—as long as it is 100 percent fruit juice— is another option.

- Discourage them from choosing soda, fruit drinks, iced tea, lemonade, and similar beverages, unless they are sweetened with noncaloric sweeteners or unsweetened.

- Always carry fruit with you as a snack or as a side item for meals out.

7

Healthier Drinking Out— Nonalcoholic Beverages

When you place your order at a restaurant, you'll almost always face the question, "What do you want to drink?" What to drink—both nonalcoholic and alcoholic—may be nothing but an afterthought to you. Once you realize how many calories you quickly rack up from regular soda, fruit drinks, lemonade and fancy coffee concoctions, you may change your thinking. The question, "What do you want to drink?" deserves a moment or two of contemplation. (Note: See Chapter 8 for alcoholic beverages.)

More Beverage Options, More Volume

Just as the variety of foods available at restaurants has expanded dramatically in recent years, so has the variety of beverages. In fact, the new bounty of beverages has expanded to an even greater degree in supermarkets and convenience stores— carbonated beverages alone usually occupy an entire supermarket aisle, even in superstores.

As the variety has grown, so have the quantities that are served in restaurants. In some fast-food restaurants, a single-serving beverage can top 32 ounces (a full quart). At coffee shops, many drinks are served in portions as large as 20 ounces, or more than two cups.

Beverages Available at Most Restaurants

- Water (tap or bottled)
- Carbonated soft drinks (regular and diet)
- Fruit drinks, punches, and lemonade (regular and diet)
- Fruit juices (usually orange and apple, but more if a full bar is available)
- Milk (whole, lowfat, and/or nonfat)
- Coffee (black, sweetened and/or with cream, and some sugary coffee "drinks")
- Tea (unsweetened, diet, and sweetened)

Beverages: An Obesity Culprit

In 2006, a proposed beverage guidance system created by leading obesity experts was published in the *American Journal of Clinical Nutrition*. Check out these statistics: The experts found that on average, American adults drink 230 calories from beverages daily, but almost half of American adults drink 500 calories a day. In addition to drinking more beverages with calorie-containing sweeteners, Americans are drinking these beverages in much larger portions. The average serving size grew from 14 to 21 ounces between 1977 and 1996.

Beverages Fill Out, Not Up

Studies show that beverages don't satisfy your appetite like solid foods do. Unfortunately, people do not decrease their solid-food caloric intake to compensate for the extra calories they receive in the form of beverages. Some experts believe that drinking calorie-laden beverages is the quickest way to pack on pounds. See how easily you can shave calories by changing your choice of beverages in the chart below.

Change Your Beverages to Shave Calories

Higher Calorie Beverages		Low-Calorie and Noncaloric Beverages		
Beverage*	Calories	Beverage*	Calories	Calories Saved
Regular Soda	96	Diet Soda	0	96
Coffee with Sugar (2 tsp) and Half-and-Half (2 tbsp)	70	Coffee with No Sugar or Sugar Substitute and 2 Percent Milk (2 tbsp)	18	52
Sweetened Iced Tea	90	Unsweetened or Diet Iced Tea	0	90
Milk (whole)	150	Nonfat Milk	90	60
Fruit Punch (Sweetened)	200	Water	0	200
Lemonade (Sweetened)	250	Lemonade (Diet)	0	250

*All 8-ounce servings. However, keep in mind that with the exception of milk, few beverages are actually provided in 8-ounce servings. Most beverage servings are much bigger.

Key Health Message: Think Before You Drink

The Dietary Guidelines suggest that you drink "beverages with little added sugars or caloric sweeteners to reduce calorie intake and achieve nutrition goals and weight control." Of course, it is also the Dietary Guidelines' recommendation to trim added sugars and calories without nutrients wherever you can. The guidelines recommend that you choose beverages that are either noncaloric or packed with nutrients. The *American Journal of Clinical Nutrition's* proposed beverage guidance system echoes this advice even more pointedly, suggesting that at least two-thirds of what you drink every day should be noncaloric beverages. Below is a list of suggested beverages.

1. Water, and lots of it.

2. Unsweetened (or sugar-substitute sweetened) coffee or tea. If you must add milk, use the nonfat kind.

3. Milk, but make it nonfat whenever possible. Milk is an excellent source of calcium, vitamin D, and other vitamins and minerals.

4. Fruit juice—and only 100 percent juice—is an option that provides nutrients along with calories. When you choose a fruit juice, make sure it is not actually a fruit drink, punch, cocktail, or "ade" (such as lemonade), which are generally sweetened with sugar or high-fructose corn syrup.

5. "Diet" carbonated soft drinks sweetened with low-calorie sweeteners. Say no to regular soda, no matter how old you are.

Just How Much?

For many years, experts preached that the right amount of beverage intake per day was eight individual 8-ounce servings daily, but this recommendation is now passé. In 2004, the Institute of Medicine (IOM), a government health advisory organization, reported that fluid needs vary widely based on many factors, including climate and food choices. Most people stay hydrated by letting their thirst guide them. When it's warm outside or you are exercising, you need to drink more to stay hydrated. IOM recommends that the proper baseline hydration requirement for women is 91 ounces a day and for men, 125 ounces a day—between 12 and 16 8-ounce servings daily.

Tips and Tactics to Tally Fewer Calories from Beverages

Coffee

Numerous chain restaurants from coast to coast make coffee drinks the centerpiece of their menus. At most of these establishments, baked items and sandwiches are little more than an afterthought. The international leader in the field is Starbucks Coffee, of course, but Dunkin' Donuts and Caribou Coffee also have a significant presence in certain regions of the U.S. Of course, there are also plenty of other local and regional coffee-shop chains.

The debates about the health benefits of coffee in general and caffeine in particular have been raging for decades. Still, there is no absolute conclusion. Some studies that observed health and eating behaviors of adults have noted some benefits of drinking coffee, such as a reduced risk of type 2 diabetes, Parkinson's disease, and some cancers. There is also no conclusion about the health benefits or risks of caffeine. Some people can't tolerate caffeine at any time of the day; others can handle it until mid-afternoon; and still others can drink a cup of java at night before going to sleep with absolutely no effect.

Whether you go for the kick of caffeine or prefer decaf, coffee is a noncaloric beverage. That's true whether it's a regular brew or a deep, dark espresso. The calories creep in when scoops of sugar (16 calories per teaspoon) and spoonfuls of half-and-half (40 calories per ounce, or 2 tablespoons) are stirred in. Even more calories tally up when flavored syrups, whipped cream, or such delights as caramel topping are added. Check out the totals in the table below.

Item	Amount	Calories	Carb (g)	Fat (g)
Mocha Frappuccino Blended Coffee (Starbucks)	24 oz	500	82	17
Iced Caramel Macchiato (Starbucks)	24 oz	330	49	8
Caramel Swirl Latte (Dunkin' Donuts)	10 oz	230	37	7
Iced Latte with Sugar (Dunkin' Donuts)	16 oz	170	23	7
Espresso Cooler (Caribou Coffee)	24 oz	250	31	13
Campfire Mocha (Caribou Coffee)	24 oz	710	121	19

Clearly, the larger sizes of some coffee concoctions contain more calories than many people should eat in an entire meal—let alone sipping a drink.

It's easy enough to lighten the calorie, carbohydrate and fat-gram load in coffee. Because the drinks are made to order, you can get it exactly as you want it. Start with unadulterated coffee and avoid the sugary blends that some of the drinks are made from. Next, choose a lowfat or no-fat creamer, such as lowfat or nonfat milk. Starting in 2007, Starbucks Coffee automatically uses lowfat milk unless customers request a lower- (nonfat) or higher- (whole milk or half-and-half) fat option. All Starbucks outlets also offer soy milk for people who are lactose-intolerant, do not eat animal products, or simply prefer its taste. Be sure to request lowfat and/or calcium-fortified soy milk if that is your preference.

Feel free to enjoy flavoring in your coffee—as long as it is sugar-free or low-calorie. Skip the half-and-half, the whipped cream, and the rich toppings; they load on calories and saturated fat. Sweeten your brew with a noncaloric sweetener—yellow, pink, or blue—instead of sugar. If all the items you add to your beverage are low-calorie, you can indulge in a large size. However, if you must occasionally splurge on a higher-calorie coffee drink, order a small portion.

In the past, espresso, a rich, dark, and thick coffee native to Italy, was usually served in a tiny portion (about 3 ounces) to finish off a meal or to sip with a sweet treat. Today, espresso is the base of myriad coffee drinks, such as cappuccino, latte, and iced coffee. Espresso is a strong coffee, which explains why it is often served in a demitasse cup with a twist of lemon and sugar cubes to cut its bitter taste. Like all other coffee, it is noncaloric until other ingredients are mixed in.

Tea

Tea is one of the most widely consumed beverages in the world, but in the past (and to the this day outside the United States) it has mainly been consumed as a hot beverage. Today, tea drinkers can choose from an endless list of options: green, black, herbal, fruit, or white teas—just to name a few—served hot or cold. You will frequently encounter varieties of tea mixed with caloric sweeteners in sandwich shops and take-out ethnic restaurants where you can purchase bottled or canned drinks. The Coca-Cola Company has introduced Enviga, a tea drink it claims will burn calories.

Don't forget chai, which has become popular in large part because of its arrival on coffee-shop menus across the country.

Chai, the word for tea on the Indian subcontinent, is traditionally made with rich black tea, whole milk, a combination of various spices, and a calorie-containing sweetener. Naturally, this means that chai usually contains a hefty amount of calories as well. Check out the numbers for chai and other sweetened teas in the chart below.

Item	Amount	Calories	Carb (g)	Fat (g)
Chai Tea with 2 percent milk—hot or iced (Caribou Coffee)	24 oz	270	46	5
Chai Iced Tea Latte (Starbucks)	24 oz	350	55	6
Black Shaken Tea and Lemonade (Starbucks)	24 oz	190	50	0
Raspberry Sweetened Iced Tea (Dunkin' Donuts)	16 oz	90	22	0
English Breakfast Tea with Milk and Sugar (Dunkin' Donuts)	10 oz	70	14	1
Asia Plum Tea (Arizona)	20 oz (bottle)	175	45	0

In coffee shops, there are usually quite a few blends of black tea, such as Earl Grey, English Breakfast, and Darjeeling. Most are available with or without caffeine. In addition to these standard choices, there are usually several caffeine-free herbal, fruit, and/or spiced options, such as chamomile, lemon lift, raspberry, or orange and spice. Upscale restaurants often offer their patrons an extensive variety of hot teas presented in a wooden box.

The debates about the health benefits of tea are similar to those of coffee. Since almost all of the black teas contain caffeine, it is naturally part of the debate as well, but cup-for-cup, teas contain less caffeine than coffee. Some of the research on tea has found that it may benefit the immune system, reducing the frequency of such illnesses as prostate cancer and psoriasis. Many remain unconvinced that tea offers significant health benefits.

Although unsweetened hot or iced tea is noncaloric, you should be very careful with tea-based beverages that contain sweeteners or creamers and follow the guidelines given in the *Coffee* section above. If you purchase iced tea in a bottle or can, carefully read the label and make sure your choice is noncaloric.

Milk

Today, almost all restaurants include milk among their beverage choices. Nearly everyone in America could benefit from drinking more milk. On average, most American children and adults do not consume enough calcium. Milk consumption has dramatically decreased over the last few decades, perhaps because the spectrum of available beverages has grown.

Most restaurants offer whole and lowfat (2 percent) cow's milk. It's much less common to find nonfat milk. If it is available, choose nonfat milk; if not, choose lowfat. An 8-ounce serving of nonfat milk has 90 calories, and the same amount of whole milk has 150 calories. The extra calories in whole and lowfat milk have no nutritional benefit, but it adds a lot more saturated fat and cholesterol. Soy milk is showing up on more menus these days, but it is consistently found only in coffee shops. Read more about beverage choices for children in Chapter 6.

Fruit Juice

Fruit juices are usually available at restaurants that serve breakfast, and most fast-food restaurants stock orange juice as well (McDonald's restaurants also offer juice boxes with their kids' meals). A sit-down restaurant with a full bar should offer an array of fruit juices used as mixers in alcoholic drinks, including orange, grapefruit, tomato, and pineapple juice.

In reasonable serving sizes (4 to 8 ounces), fruit and vegetable juices are a healthy vitamin- and mineral-dense beverage choice. However, the most common serving sizes found in breakfast and sandwich shops are 12- to 16-ounce bottles, which adds as much as 240 calories to your daily consumption. Since that size beverage is comparable to a single 4-ounce serving of fruit, you are much better off choosing a whole-fruit alternative. Both the Dietary Guidelines and the *American Journal of Clinical Nutrition's* proposed beverage guidance system encourage people to eat whole fruit, which provides volume and fiber, instead of sipping fruit juice.

Smoothies

As consumers demand more quick meals and snacks, many restaurants are whipping up smoothies as an ideal on-the-go meal substitute. These frothy drinks can be made from a mixture of healthy ingredients, such as lowfat milk or yogurt, and pieces of real fruit. Unfortunately, most are blends of a few healthy ingredients and many fruit-flavored syrups and concentrates, and they are not suitable as meal replacements because beverages do not satisfy the same way solid food does.

Smoothies are generally served in unnecessarily large portions. Because of this, whether or not they are healthy, they tend to be high in calories. Even a small (16-ounce) Dunkin' Donuts smoothie has 360 calories. Most of the calories in smoothies are from carbohydrates—for example, the Dunkin' Donuts smoothie has over 100 grams of carbohydrates. The smoothies from Jamba Juice, another leading chain, have similar calorie and carbohydrate counts.

If you want a smoothie as a special treat, find a restaurant that makes them with milk or yogurt and fresh fruit only. Control your portions by sharing the smoothie with one or two dining companions. Consider your small-portion smoothie to be a sweet treat or snack instead of a meal replacement.

Carbonated Soft Drinks

Sodas, soft drinks, and pop—what you call it probably depends on where you live—are frequently consumed with restaurant foods. Fast-food restaurants are particularly focused on soft drinks; in fact, until fairly recently fast-food chains KFC, Pizza Hut, and Taco Bell were owned by a unit of PepsiCo. Soft drinks are usually served fountain-style in restaurants because fountain setups maximize profit margin: A 32-ounce serving of soda that costs you nearly two dollars costs the restaurant a few pennies. Most restaurants offer regular and diet cola and at least one citrus-flavored soda, such as 7-Up or Sprite. Sandwich shops that sell carbonated soda by the can or bottle often have a wider selection, including root beer, cream soda, and other flavors.

During the past few decades, regular soda sold in the U.S. has been sweetened with high-fructose corn syrup (HFCS). HFCS replaced cane sugar in most sweet beverages and in thousands of other processed foods because a combination of tariffs on sugar imports and government subsidies on corn production make corn syrup a far cheaper sweetener. Health advocates have been particularly vocal about HFCS in recent years, connecting the rise of HFCS to the rise of obesity in America. However, the science on this issue is still questionable.

Diet soda is also widely available. The noncaloric sweeteners used in diet soda have changed over the last several decades. Before the 1980s, almost all diet soda was sweetened with saccharin. Today, most fountain diet sodas are sweetened with a combination of aspartame and saccharin, and cans or bottles of diet soda are usually sweetened with either aspartame or sucralose.

Avoid regular soda. It's nothing more than empty calories, and a lot of them: A 20-ounce bottle of soda contains about 250 calories. If you must have the fizz, choose diet soda with no calories. While there's nothing nutritionally redeeming about diet soda either, at least you won't be consuming any calories.

Fruit Drinks (Carbonated and Uncarbonated)

Most fruit drink makers like to make a big deal about the nutritional value of their drinks. Unless they are made with 100 percent fruit juice, they probably don't have much. Fruit drinks may be uncarbonated, such as fruit punch and fruit "ades," like lemonade. Others, like fruit-flavored seltzers, are carbonated. Both types of beverages are sweetened with high-fructose corn syrup, just like soda, and they provide no redeeming nutritional benefits.

You find these beverages frequently sold in sandwich, bagel, and coffee shops. The usual serving size is a 16- or 20-ounce bottle. They are also served at fast-food fountains, and with the exception of an occasional diet lemonade drink, the fountains usually don't offer a diet alternative to fruit drinks.

However, convenience and grocery stores usually carry diet alternatives to these fruit drinks. If you choose a fruit drink, carefully inspect its Nutrition Facts label. Look for a drink that contains less than 10 calories per serving.

As with all other beverages, be aware that the Nutrition Facts labels for beverages usually specify an eight-ounce serving size. If you plan to drink a 20-ounce serving, make sure you calculate the beverage's calories correctly.

Water (Carbonated or Uncarbonated)

Last, but most important, is cheap, plentiful, accessible, noncaloric, and healthy water. The good news is that the popularity of bottled water has made it more readily available than ever before. Nearly any restaurant you enter—from fast-food to sandwich shops to fine restaurants—offers bottled water.

It's worth mentioning that tap water, which is usually free, is usually just as tasty as bottled water and in many cases is better for you: Unlike tap water, most bottled water does not contain fluoride, which is extremely beneficial for dental health. Many bottled waters are nothing more than filtered tap water. To add some flavor to your water, request a slice of lemon or lime. Kids can make their own lemonade with lemon wedges and noncaloric sweeteners.

Waters with some fizz to them are also widely available. Carbonated mineral water and club soda are both noncaloric, and a slice of lemon or lime or a splash of fruit juice can jazz up these beverages. Note that tonic water, which is usually available at restaurants with full-service bars, does contain calories.

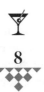

8

Healthier Drinking Out— Alcoholic Beverages

In sit-down restaurants that offer beer, wine, and/or a full complement of distilled beverages, the first question you'll probably be asked is, "What can I bring you to drink?" The restaurant's hope is that you'll order an alcoholic beverage—one of the highest profit areas in the restaurant business. Since most alcoholic beverages are loaded with calories and can negatively impact your health in other ways, the question deserves careful thought. (Note: Read Chapter 7 for a discussion of nonalcoholic beverages.)

Alcohol's Pluses

Many researchers have sought to find health benefits to consuming alcohol. Does moderate consumption of alcohol provide health benefits? At this point, it appears that light to moderate (one to two drinks per day) alcohol consumption can decrease the risk of type 2 diabetes, heart disease, and stroke. Alcohol has also been found to increase insulin sensitivity, which can lower blood glucose levels and improve other health parameters. Do some alcoholic beverages provide more benefit than others? The answer appears to be no.

If you don't currently drink alcohol, don't start just for the health benefits. There are many other, more effective ways to get and stay healthy, such as eating wisely and increasing your level of physical activity. Most people drink alcohol to relax and socialize, which is why it's more common to drink alcohol when dining out than when eating at home.

Alcohol's Minuses

Calories. The calories in alcohol are a big minus, and alcohol's calories provide practically no nutrition. The calories from alcohol can add up quickly: A 12-ounce beer contains 150 calories, a shot of distilled liquor contains 100 calories, and a five-ounce glass of wine contains 150 calories. If shedding weight is your goal, you'll need to moderate your intake of alcohol or abstain altogether—you simply can't afford the calories.

Safety. We can't discuss alcohol consumption and dining out without mentioning drinking and driving. Awareness of the dangers of drinking and driving has increased dramatically in recent years. The bottom line is that people should not drink and drive. Alcohol slows physical and mental reactions, and it impairs judgment. Drinking and driving endangers your health and the health of those around you.

Health. Drinking excessive amounts of alcohol can cause or be a risk factor for liver diseases, such as cirrhosis; high blood pressure; cancers of the gastrointestinal tract, such as the stomach; other cancers; and strokes. Women who are pregnant, breastfeeding, or planning to become pregnant are encouraged to avoid alcohol altogether, and people who have pancreatitis, a high level of triglycerides, or have abused alcohol in the past should also avoid it.

How Much Is Too Much?

The Dietary Guidelines recommend drinking no more than a moderate amount of alcohol in a single day. Moderate drinking is clearly defined as one serving of alcohol for women and two servings for men per day.

Develop Your Alcoholic Beverage Plan

Consider when enjoying an alcoholic beverage is particularly important to you—or if it is important at all. Perhaps you'll decide to drink alcohol only when you dine out on the weekends, or during one or two restaurant meals per week. If you enjoy alcohol and plan to integrate it into your lifelong healthy eating plan, start that plan today.

Tips to Limit Alcohol

- Never drink alcohol without another noncaloric beverage, such as water, by its side. Quench your thirst with the noncaloric beverage and sip your alcoholic beverage slowly—it will last much longer, and you will consume less.
- At what point during a meal do you enjoy a drink most? While you wait for your food? While you enjoy your meal? Or as an after-dinner drink? Order your alcoholic beverage at the point when you will enjoy it most.
- Order alcohol in small quantities. Unless you have enough people in your party to share an entire bottle (at least four people), order wine by the glass. If you are ordering beer, specify a 12-ounce serving instead of a pint.

Alcoholic Beverages

Beers

There are probably thousands of different beers available in American restaurants today. You can order a Singha in most Thai restaurants, a Dos Equis in a Mexican spot, a Bud in a local bar and grill, or a Sapporo in a sushi bar. Beer is a brewed and fermented drink. Most beers are blends of malted barley and other starches that are flavored with hops, but flavors can vary widely. Although they may taste very different, most beers have the same caloric content: about 150 calories for a 12-ounce serving. Light beer is not exactly "diet" beer: Unlike noncaloric diet sodas, light beers contain about a third fewer calories than regular beer, at 100 calories per 12-ounce serving.

Wines

Any wine—red, white, or rosé; domestic, French, or Italian—contains about 150 calories per five-ounce serving. Exercise portion control with wine by ordering it by the half-bottle or the glass at the point during the meal when you will enjoy it most.

Another calorie-conscious strategy is ordering a wine spritzer, which is a mixture of wine, club soda, and a twist of lemon or lime. Ask the bartender to mix yours as half wine and half club soda instead of the usual mix: three-quarters wine and one-quarter soda. You'll cut your calorie consumption in half as well.

Champagnes and Other Sparkling Wines

Champagnes and sparkling wines contain about 20 percent more calories than most wines depending on their dryness ("dry" means "less sweet"). The drier the wine, the higher the calories. Only sparkling wines from the Champagne region of France can be called champagne. Many restaurants that serve brunch include mimosas—a calorie-packed mix of sparkling wine and orange juice—with the meal.

Distilled Beverages

Rum, gin, vodka, and whiskey are all classified as distilled spirits, or "hard liquor." A single serving of each contains about the same number of calories—about 100 calories per 1.5-ounce serving of 80-proof liquor. Many people believe that sweeter distilled spirits, such as rum and bourbon, are higher in calories, but all distilled spirits are the same.

If hard liquor is what you prefer, enjoy it in moderation. Distilled spirits are often mixed with other high-calorie non-alcoholic liquids, such as fruit juices, tonic water, milk or cream, or syrups. A 5-ounce serving of a piña colada, which contains rum, coconut cream, and pineapple juice, has 250 calories. Many other mixed drinks also include other high-calorie liqueurs. Limit your intake of drinks that combine distilled spirits, liqueurs, fruit juice, regular soda, tonic water, or cream. Order distilled spirits on the rocks with a splash of water, club soda, or diet soda.

Liqueurs and Brandies

Liqueurs, cordials, and brandies constitute another category of alcoholic beverages. Liqueurs and cordials, including such well-known brands as Kahlua, Amaretto di Saronno, Grand Marnier, and Chambord, are served straight-up or on the rocks as after-dinner drinks or in combination with other distilled spirits in a mixed drink (see the *Distilled Beverages* section above). Brandies are distilled wines or fermented fruit juices, and the most commonly ordered brandy is cognac. Liqueurs, cordials, and brandies contain about 150 calories per 1.5-ounce serving, a substantial number of calories for a small amount of liquid.

An easy way to keep your calories down and enjoy liqueurs is to order a liqueur-based coffee drink, such as Irish coffee or Kahlua and coffee, for dessert. A shot of liqueur in black coffee makes a delicious drink that can be slowly sipped—but be sure to tell your server to hold the whipped cream and sugar. The liqueur in a coffee drink will satisfy any sweet tooth all by itself. As your dining companions are downing high-calorie confections, you can sip your 150-calorie, nonfat dessert. Cheers!

9

Breakfast—From Bagels to Bakeries to Brunch

During the hustle-bustle of the workweek, you might find yourself grabbing breakfast at a corner coffee shop or national coffee chain. You might select a jumbo muffin, scone, or bagel with cream cheese and a steaming cup of hot coffee or cappuccino to eat in your car or at your desk. Or maybe you choose to visit the drive-through window at a fast-food chain and buy an egg, sausage, and cheese sandwich with an orange juice. On weekends, you might order a pile of pancakes or a whipped-cream-and-syrup-topped waffle at the local pancake house or an all-you-can-eat champagne brunch at a downtown hotel or countryside retreat.

Over the last two decades, breakfast foods have changed dramatically, and more people than ever before eat breakfast out or grab it to-go and eat it on the run. Our frenetic lifestyles have created a need for handheld breakfast foods that you can eat on-the-go or in the car. This need has given rise to the fast-food breakfast sandwich—a biscuit, English muffin, bagel, or croissant filled with as little as butter or cream cheese or as much as eggs, cheese, and breakfast meats, such as sausage, bacon, or ham. Chain coffee shops, such as Starbucks and Caribou Coffee, serve plain and gussied-up java, scones, muffins, and bagels to their hungry morning crowds; not wanting to be left out, the independent shops have followed suit as well. Hundreds of chain and independent bagel shops have opened as well, specializing in coffee, bagels, and bagel sandwiches. Doughnut shops, such as Dunkin' Donuts and Krispy Kreme, have tried to keep pace with the coffee shops and now serve bagels, muffins, and breakfast sandwiches.

Nutrition Snapshot

The following nutrition snapshot is intended to provide you with nutrition numbers for a handful of common menu items served for breakfast at doughnut and bagel shops, sit-down restaurants, and fast-food restaurants. You'll see numbers that range from mind-blowing to healthy. Use them to educate yourself about the nutrition facts of your current breakfast choices. You may just find yourself changing your favorite orders.

Menu Item	Calories	Carbohydrate (g)	Fat (g)	Saturated Fat (g)	*Trans* Fat (g)	Sodium (mg)
Coffee and Coffee Drinks (Hot)						
Regular, Black—12 oz	8	2	0	0	0	6
Caffe Latte (Nonfat Milk)—12 oz (Starbucks)	100	15	1	0	0	120
Caffe Mocha (with Whipped Cream & Nonfat Milk)—12 oz (Starbucks)	230	34	8	4	0	110
Cappuccino (with Sugar)—10 oz (Dunkin' Donuts)	130	21	5	3	0	65
Cappuccino (Nonfat)—16 oz (Einstein Bagels)	150	19	7	4.5	0	190
Espresso—1.5 oz (Einstein Bagels)	1	0	0	0	0	0

The plainer, the better. If you must use a creamer, use lowfat or nonfat milk. Skip the high-calorie sweeteners and syrups.

Menu Item	Calories	Carbohy-drate (g)	Fat (g)	Saturated Fat (g)	*Trans* Fat (g)	Sodium (mg)
Coffee and Coffee Drinks (Cold)						
Coffee Coolatta (with Cream)—16 oz (Dunkin' Donuts)	350	40	22	14	0	65
Coffee Coolatta (2 Percent Milk)—16 oz (Dunkin' Donuts)	190	41	2	1.5	0	80
Iced Latte (Nonfat)—16 oz (Einstein Bagels)	90	12	0	0	0	130
Iced Mocha (Lowfat)—16 oz (Einstein Bagels)	180	30	3	2	0	115
The plainer, the better. If you must use a creamer, use lowfat or nonfat milk. Skip the high-calorie sweeteners and syrups.						
Fruit and Juice						
Orange Juice—10 oz	140	34	0	0	0	5
Apple Juice—10 oz	125	33	0	0	0	24
Fresh Fruit Cup—8 oz	110	25	0	0	0	10
Make sure it is 100 percent fruit juice. Skip the fruit punches and fruit drinks. A healthy choice.						
Cereals						
Cold: Raisin Bran—1 cup	190	45	1.5	0	0	350
Cold: Cheerios—1 cup	110	22	2	0	0	280
Hot: Oatmeal, Plain (Denny's)	100	18	2	0	0	270
Hot: Grits—4 oz (Shoney's)	105	11	6	1	na	158
A healthy choice with nonfat or lowfat milk and fruit.						
Breakfast Entrées						
Eggs Benedict (Denny's)	760	52	40	15	.5	2400
French Toast Platter (Denny's)	1261	110	79	30	0	2490
Ham 'n' Cheddar Omelet (Denny's)	595	5	47	16	.5	1200
Skip or split 'em.						

Menu Item	Calories	Carbohy-drate (g)	Fat (g)	Saturated Fat (g)	*Trans* Fat (g)	Sodium (mg)
Hotcakes—3 plain (Denny's)	491	95	7	1	0	1820
Buttermilk Pancakes—3 (IHOP)	420	82	5	1	na	1350
Waffle—1 (IHOP)	310	37	15	4	na	380

Split 'em. These are probably enough for two.

Bagels

Menu Item	Calories	Carbohy-drate (g)	Fat (g)	Saturated Fat (g)	*Trans* Fat (g)	Sodium (mg)
Cinnamon raisin (Manhattan Bagels)	340	76	1	0	na	570
Everything (Dunkin' Donuts)	370	67	6	.5	0	650
Honey Whole Wheat (Einstein Bagels)	360	64	1	0	na	510
Sesame (Tim Horton's)	270	53	3	0	0	430
Flaxseed (Tim Horton's)	290	53	5	.5	0	520
Blueberry (Dunkin' Donuts)	330	66	3	.5	0	600

A reasonable lowfat choice, but remember that they are high in carbs and calories. Consider half or two-thirds of a bagel. Order regular or light spread on the side, and spread it very thinly.

Doughnuts

Menu Item	Calories	Carbohy-drate (g)	Fat (g)	Saturated Fat (g)	*Trans* Fat (g)	Sodium (mg)
Cinnamon Cake (Dunkin' Donuts)	330	34	20	5	4	340
Glazed Cake (Dunkin' Donuts)	350	41	19	5	4	340
Traditional Cake (Krispy Kreme)	230	20	13	3	4	320
Glazed Yeast (Dunkin' Donuts)	180	25	8	1.5	4	250
Glazed Lemon Filled (Krispy Kreme)	290	35	16	4	5	135

Eat just once in a while. Healthwise, they're nothing to brag about, but you can eat just one, since the portions are small. As you can see, some of the choices are better than others.

Menu Item	Calories	Carbohydrate (g)	Fat (g)	Saturated Fat (g)	*Trans* Fat (g)	Sodium (mg)
Muffins						
Honey Raisin Bran (Dunkin' Donuts)	480	79	15	2.5	0	480
Blueberry (Dunkin' Donuts)	470	73	17	3	0	500
Poppyseed (Einstein Bagels)	350	79	2	0	0	680
Carrot Whole Wheat (Tim Horton's)	400	55	19	3	0	660
Cranberry Lowfat (Tim Horton's)	290	62	3	.5	0	750

Consider splitting into two breakfasts. The calorie content in the lowfat muffin is more reasonable.

Croissants						
Plain (Dunkin' Donuts)	330	37	18	5	7	270
Cheese (Tim Horton's)	370	37	20	7	5	410
Butter (Tim Horton's)	340	38	18	5	5	380

Skip 'em all. They're loaded with fat.

Breakfast Sandwiches						
Sausage Biscuit (Shoney's)	539	42	34	9	na	1655
Skip 'em.						
Sausage Biscuit (Burger King)	390	28	26	7	5	1410
Skip 'em.						
Sausage, Egg, and Cheese McGriddle (McDonald's)	560	48	32	12	0	1360
Skip 'em.						
Egg McMuffin (McDonald's)	300	30	12	5	0	820
OK.						
Bacon, Egg, and Cheese Biscuit (McDonald's)	520	43	30	13	0	1520
Skip 'em.						
Breaded Pork Chop Biscuit (Hardee's)	690	48	42	8	na	1330
Skip 'em.						
Egg, Ham, and Cheese Bagel (Manhattan Bagels)	550	74	15	8	na	1710
OK.						

Menu Item	Calories	Carbohy-drate (g)	Fat (g)	Saturated Fat (g)	*Trans* Fat (g)	Sodium (mg)
Breakfast Sides						
Bacon—4 pieces (Denny's)	162	1	18	5	0	640
Bacon—3 pieces (Shoney's)	120	0	11	5	na	405
Ham (Denny's)	85	6	3	2	0	1700
Sausage—4 pieces (Denny's)	354	0	32	12	0	944
Sausage Patty—1 piece (Shoney's)	209	0	18	6	na	74
Split the order, and only order these once in a while.						

The Menu Profile

Most people think of breakfast as the lightest meal of the day, especially during the work week. However, doughnuts, bagels with a thick layer of cream cheese, and breakfast sandwiches contain a lot more calories than you think— and a load of fat. The challenge is to find quick and easy breakfast choices that are low in fat and calories and fall into the harder-to-fulfill food groups, such as whole grains, fruits, and dairy foods. Consider choosing half of a bagel or muffin, a piece of fruit and/or a hard boiled egg, a whole-grain English muffin with a slice of lowfat cheese and a piece of fruit, or a bowl of hot or cold cereal and nonfat milk topped with fruit.

Most importantly, take a realistic approach: Shoot for the goal of consuming 20 to 30 percent of your daily calories at breakfast. Keep the carbohydrates up and the protein (meats, primarily, since most breakfast meats are particularly high in fat) and fat down. You'll want to save the protein and fat for lunch and dinner. If you load up on protein in the morning by eating a two-

or three-egg omelet with cheese, it will be hard to limit protein later in the day. (Not to mention the excess saturated fat and cholesterol in a three-egg omelet with cheese!)

The best that can be said about "all-you-can-eat" breakfast or brunch buffets is that they should be avoided. If the restaurant also offers menu service during the buffet, you are safe: You can always order a healthier choice while your dining companions indulge in the buffet. Otherwise, choose a different restaurant.

If you absolutely must visit a brunch buffet, a few simple watchwords will help you keep the calories down.

1. Take an initial survey of the situation. Peruse the buffet and check out the foods that are offered. Plan what you will eat, and in what quantity.
2. Try a plate of fresh fruit or salad as a first course to take the edge off your appetite.
3. If many items on the buffet appeal to you, take very small quantities of them. Another plus—you will not waste food.
4. Drink plenty of noncaloric fluids, eat slowly, and enjoy the relaxing environment and the company of your dining companions.
5. Burn the additional calories with extra exercise before or after you've digested the brunch.

Coffee

It's not just plain java any longer. Today, the choice of coffees is greater than ever. Hot coffees include regular, decaffeinated, espresso, café au lait, cappuccino, café latte, and café mocha, to name a few. More variations are created every day. Serving sizes vary, too: You'll encounter everything from a simple cup of coffee to Starbucks' largest size, the venti (fun fact: "venti" is Italian for 20—as in 20 ounces).

That's not even to mention the slew of cold coffee drinks now available in coffee, doughnut, and bagel shops. Starbucks has made the Frappuccino and the Caramel Macchiatto famous, and Dunkin' Donuts offers its Coolattas. The syrups, whipped cream, and other high-fat ingredients in these cold drinks—as well as the huge portion sizes—escalate the calories and fat grams. When it comes to coffee drinks, the plainer, the better. Choose lowfat or nonfat milk and low-carbohydrate and low-calorie sweeteners and syrups. Read more about coffee in Chapter 7.

Fruit and Juice

When you think of breakfast, you probably think of fresh orange juice. Few people are aware that a small 6-ounce glass of almost any juice contains at least 60 calories. They are healthy, nutrition-dense calories, but you are always better off eating fruit rather than drinking juice. Order grapefruit or a slice of melon, or split a bowl of fresh fruit with a dining companion.

Juice and fruit, with the exception of the occasional banana, is not usually part of the grab-and-go breakfast scene. If you do happen to find it at a convenient place, it's usually a huge portion of juice or cut fruit, and it is way overpriced. If you do order fruit or juice, split it, or take part of it home to enjoy later. If you want to save money too, get your fruit at home before you leave the house—sip on a glass of juice (4 to 8 ounces is plenty) as you get dressed or grab a piece of fruit and eat it on the way to work (bananas, apples, and dried fruit are very portable).

Cereal

Cold cereals, which are almost always available at breakfast restaurants, are appearing at more cafés these days. Thank goodness there aren't nearly as many choices there as in the super-market! A few standard choices are not sugar-coated, including cornflakes, puffed wheat, shredded wheat, rice cereals (Rice Krispies), plain bran flakes, and bran flakes with raisins. Others are highly sweetened, including Frosted Flakes, Fruit Loops, and Trix. You are best off choosing a whole-grain, high-fiber cereal. Almost all cold cereals—whether they are sugar-coated or not—have sugar, or a form of sugar, in their top four ingredients.

Hot cereals are often among the breakfast menu items at sit-down restaurants, cafeterias, and hotels. Oatmeal, the most common of the hot cereals, is a healthy choice. If you add milk, pour on the lowfat variety (nonfat milk is often hard to find in restaurants). If you have the option of topping cold or hot cereal with bananas, strawberries or raisins, go right ahead. All are healthy and add a serving of fruit to your daily intake.

Breakfast Entrées

Pancakes, French toast, and waffles are basically made from the same ingredients: flour, water, egg, sugar, and a leavening agent. Before the whipped butter and syrup are loaded on, they're not necessarily nutrition disasters, but they don't usually contain whole grains or fiber (some restaurants do list whole-wheat or whole-grain pancakes on their menus; if so, it's an excellent choice). The biggest problem is the portions—they are usually too high and/or too wide. To solve that problem, share an order, or order a "short stack" of pancakes. Ask the server to hold the butter and use only a bit of real maple syrup, or top them with fresh fruit, jam, jelly, or a noncaloric sweetener and cinnamon (especially good on French toast), and their health quotient will dramatically improve.

Eggs can be a big problem. Unfortunately, they usually come two or three at a time and are accompanied by fried breakfast potatoes, toast, and often a high-fat breakfast meat as well. Remember, you can always order à la carte; poached eggs are usually the lowest-fat option.

Probably the biggest issue with eggs is their cholesterol content—just over 200 milligrams per egg, all from the yolk. However, eggs have moderate saturated-fat content, and most people can tolerate a few eggs each week. Omelets are usually made with three eggs and contain many high-fat ingredients. You are best off sharing an omelet filled with flavorful veggies, like onions, peppers, and spinach, and a leaner meat, such as ham. If you share with a dining companion, you'll only consume half the calories, fat, and cholesterol.

You may also ask that the restaurant use an egg substitute in your omelet. Egg substitutes are mostly egg whites with some flavoring, vitamins, and color added. They are a very healthy and cholesterol-free alternative to whole eggs.

Bagels, Breads, Doughnuts, Muffins, and More

Most restaurants offer many selections from the bread category at breakfast. Some are healthy, and others are best left on the shelf. Let's start with the muffin. Today's muffins are at least twice the size of the muffins your grandmother used to bake. On average, these "mega-muffins" contain somewhere between 350–500 calories—even the lowfat varieties. If the muffin you want is enormous, only eat half of it. Save the other half for the next day, or share it. Complement the half-muffin with a piece of fruit and/or a small container of yogurt.

Bagels are bigger than ever as well. An average bagel in a bagel or coffee shop is equivalent to at least four to five slices of bread, or 350 to 450 calories. Unfortunately, most people think a bagel is equivalent to two slices of bread, or about 160 calories. Next comes several tablespoons of cream cheese: Before you know it, you've eaten 500 to 600 calories. Find a bagel shop that serves relatively small bagels, and take advantage of the lighter spreads. Always order the spread on the side, so you can choose how much to put on your bagel. Consider splitting a bagel and complementing it with fruit, a hard-boiled egg, or yogurt.

Croissants, biscuits, and doughnuts are loaded with fat, and therefore they contain excess calories. Keep these on your once-in-a-while list. Healthier breakfast breads, which contain little or no fat, are bread, bagels, and English muffins. Choose whole-grain varieties whenever possible, and always be careful about what you load on that bread. Request that it be served dry, with the spreads on the side. Keep margarine, butter, cream cheese, and other fats you spread on the bread to a minimum. Use low-sugar preserves, jams, or jellies instead.

Breakfast Sandwiches

Unfortunately, America's desire for quick and easy-to-hold breakfast sandwiches is here to stay. The sandwiches are usually a bagel, biscuit, croissant, or English muffin filled with one or more high-fat items: eggs, cheese, bacon, sausage, ham, or even fried chicken. If you must eat a breakfast sandwich, order one served on an English muffin or bagel, and select a leaner meat, like ham or Canadian bacon.

Breakfast Sides

Breakfast sides often add a shocking amount of fat and calories to breakfast. The usual breakfast meats are bacon, sausage, ham, and Canadian bacon. Opt for the leaner ham or Canadian bacon. If a restaurant offers a lean chicken, turkey, or meatless sausage, opt for it instead. Breakfast potatoes, whether they are called hash browns or home fries, are another example of taking a great food—potatoes—and adding unnecessary fat and sodium to them during the cooking process. The fast-food varieties of breakfast potatoes are usually deep-fried (instead of pan-fried) and therefore derive even more of their calories from fat.

Many restaurants now offer yogurt and cottage cheese as side orders. Both can be healthy additions to any breakfast. Enjoy them with fruit or breakfast breads. It is often wise to order the sides à la carte, but be warned: It can get expensive. Healthier sides include fresh fruit, yogurt, cottage cheese, whole-wheat toast, or a bagel. If you decide to share an order of pancakes, French toast, or waffles, order yogurt and fresh fruit à la carte as toppings.

Typical Menu: Breakfast or Brunch

☼ *Indicates preferred choices*

Fruits and Juices

☼ **Juice, small** (orange, grapefruit, apple, cranberry, tomato)
☼ **Grapefruit half**
☼ **Fresh fruit cup** (Note: The serving is often enough for two to share.)
☼ **Sliced melon**
☼ **Fruit platter with yogurt or cottage cheese** (Note: A fruit platter is often enough for three people to share.)

Cereals

☼ **Cold cereal** (corn flakes, Special K)
☼ **Cold cereal** (bran flakes, shredded wheat)
Cold cereal (Frosted Flakes, Fruit Loops, Trix)
☼ **Granola** (natural, oat-based cereal filled with nuts and grains)
☼ **Hot cereal** (oatmeal, Cream of Wheat)

Pancakes, French Toast, and Waffles

Request that the butter and syrup should be served on the side, and plan to share these servings with a dining companion.

✿ **Buttermilk pancakes**, stack of 3, large

✿ **Silver-dollar pancakes** (10–12 small buttermilk pancakes)

✿ **Blueberry pancakes** (three large buttermilk pancakes filled with blueberries)

French toast (four slices of extra-thick bread dipped in egg batter and fried)

Belgian waffle

Eggs

✿ **Two eggs** (fried, scrambled, hard-boiled, or poached)

✿ **Egg substitute** (the serving size should be the equivalent of two eggs)

Eggs Benedict (two English muffin halves topped with Canadian bacon, poached eggs, and hollandaise sauce)

Steak and eggs (two eggs prepared to order served with an 8-ounce sirloin strip steak)

Three-Egg Omelet

Plan to share your omelet with a dining companion.

Western (contains sautéed onions and green peppers and is usually smothered in Cheddar cheese and diced ham)

Florentine (contains spinach, onions, and feta cheese and is topped with a creamy mushroom sauce)

✿ **Veggie** (contains sautéed onions, green and red peppers, mushrooms, and other vegetables; it is often also topped with Swiss cheese)

Breads/Bakery

Request that butter, margarine, jelly, jam, or any other spread be served on the side.

Plan to share large muffins or bagels with a dining companion.

Croissant (plain, almond, ham and cheese)

✿ **Muffin** (blueberry, raisin bran, carrot raisin, and perhaps a lowfat option, which is the best choice).

✿ **Bagel** (with lowfat cream cheese served on the side)

Danish pastry (choice of apple, raspberry, or cheese)

Doughnuts

✿ **Toast** (choice of white, whole-wheat, rye, or pumpernickel) (Note: It is best to select whole-wheat or other whole-grain bread.)

✿ **English muffin**

Side Orders

✿ **One egg** (fried, scrambled, hard-boiled, or poached) (Note: Hard-boiled and poached eggs are healthier choices than the other two methods of preparation.)

Bacon

Sausage (links or patties)

✿ **Ham or Canadian bacon**

Home fries

Hash browns

✿ **Cottage cheese**

✿ **Fruited or plain yogurt**

✿ **Fresh fruit cup** (Note: The usual serving is often enough for two.)

.... ◀ **"May I Take Your Order"** ▶ ····················

Low-Calorie Sample Meal

Banana, sliced
Quantity: ½
Cold or hot cereal (high-fiber
bran, oatmeal, or oat bran)
Quantity: 1 box or 1 cup
Lowfat or nonfat milk
Quantity: 1 cup

NUTRITION SUMMARY
272 calories
Carb: 48 g, 71%
Fat: 4 g, 13%
Protein: 11 g, 16%
Cholesterol: 20 mg
Sodium: 340 mg

Moderate-Calorie Sample Meal

Orange juice
Quantity: 6 oz.
Egg, poached
Quantity: 1
Bagel (cream cheese served
on the side)
Quantity: 1 small
Lowfat veggie cream cheese
Quantity: 1 tablespoon

NUTRITION SUMMARY
541 calories
Carb: 69 g, 51%
Fat: 22 g, 37%
Protein: 16 g, 12%
Cholesterol: 228 mg
Sodium: 560mg

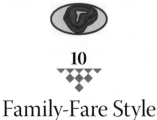

10

Family-Fare Style

Several national family-fare chains serve food from sunup to sundown, such as Cracker Barrel, Denny's, Shoney's, Bakers Square, and Bob Evans. Chili's, Bennigan's, Applebee's, Ruby Tuesday, Red Lobster, California Pizza Kitchen, The Cheesecake Factory, and T.G.I. Friday's offer menus for lunch and dinner filled with typical American foods, as well as Mexican, Chinese, and Italian favorites. These restaurants also offer entire menus of alcoholic beverages and rich desserts to accompany your meal. Family-fare cuisine also includes steak houses, such as the increasingly popular Aussie-themed Outback Steakhouse and the upscale chains Ruth's Chris and Morton's, and steak, potato and salad-bar type restaurants like Ponderosa, Steak and Ale, Sizzler, Ryan's, and Lone Star Steakhouse.

In each category of family-fare restaurants, there are also plenty of independently owned and operated dining spots. The chains and the independents have a few areas of common ground: At these outlets, you sit down and place an order, your food is brought to your table, and, generally speaking, the foods they offer are high in fat and calories. And all these restaurants certainly have one other thing in common: Their portions are HUGE!

Most family-fare restaurants serve a wide gamut of foods, from all-American options meat and potatoes, burgers and fries, and, of course, apple pie, to a multiethnic mix of Italian pastas and entrées, Chinese cashew chicken or potstickers, and Mexican fajitas or tacos. Family-fare restaurants aim to offer something for everyone—a potpourri of foods and flavors from around the world. Steak houses offer narrower menus that focus on large cuts of red meat, potatoes, and salads, and a trip or two to the salad bar.

Family-fare cuisine leaves much to be desired for the health-oriented diner. It's loaded with fat—fried mozzarella sticks, French fries, and super nachos, for example—and heavy on protein, like half-pound hamburgers, whole chicken breasts, and portions of seafood that are twice what you need. Vegetables, fruits, whole grains and dairy foods are scarce, and most vegetables are covered in butter or cheese sauces. The portions are often enough for two ore even more.

The big challenge in family-fare restaurants is to limit overeating. Family-style eating is not the norm, but it is the best way to go in these restaurants if you want to control your portions (and save money). Take advantage of soup or salad and half-sandwich combinations. Split different parts of your meal with a dining companion. Splurge with a dessert occasionally, but share it with a friend.

If you can't convince anyone to share, go it alone. Split a large dinner salad or entrée with yourself: Ask for a to-go container when you place your order and as soon as you're served, place half the meal in the container. This will reduce the amount of food in front of you from the start so you don't overeat in the end.

Nutrition Snapshot

The following nutrition snapshot is intended to provide you with the nutrition numbers for a handful of common menu items served at family-fare restaurants. You'll see nutrition numbers that range from mind-blowing to healthy. Use them to educate yourself about the nutrition makeup of your current favorite order in family-fare restaurants. If necessary, choose new, healthier favorites.

Menu Item	Calories	Carbohydrate (g)	Fat (g)	Saturated Fat (g)	*Trans* Fat (g)	Sodium (mg)
Fried Whole Onion with Dipping Sauce—1 serving (The Lone Star)	953	71	62	20	na	790
Skip this one unless you have a table full of people.						
Buffalo Wings—9 pieces (Denny's)	974	11	72	18	0	4049
Skip 'em, or have just one or two wings.						
Chicken Fingers, fried—5 pieces (Bob Evans)	650	42	36.2	6.3	.8	1505
Stick with grilled or barbecue chicken.						
Bean Soup—1 bowl (Bob Evans)	205	27	5	1.5	0	1110
A healthy bet for a starter or entrée, but it is high in sodium.						
Sirloin Steak—5 oz raw wt (Bob Evans)	403	0	27	8	0.2	637
Portion will be 4 oz cooked, a relatively small restaurant portion.						
Tenderloin Steak—9 oz. raw wt (Road House Grill)	681	0	54	na	na	125
A leaner cut of beef. You'll get about 7 ounces cooked. This portion could easily be shared with another diner.						
New York Strip Steak—12 oz (The Lone Star)	1036	0	80	32	na	210
A large piece of meat, more than enough for two. Request a smaller portion.						
Meat Loaf—1 slice (Denny's)	282	9	19	7.6	.6	1755
High in fat, saturated fat, and sodium.						
Steakhouse Strip Dinner (Denny's)	390	0	14	5	0	460
A reasonable choice.						

Menu Item	Calories	Carbohy-drate (g)	Fat (g)	Saturated Fat (g)	*Trans* Fat (g)	Sodium (mg)
Classic Burger (Denny's)	780	56	45	17	2.5	1030
Stick with grilled chicken instead.						
Barbecued Chicken—1 piece (Bob Evans)	325	22	13	3	.5	783
Remove the skin to cut out fat and calories.						
Grilled Chicken—6 oz (The Lone Star)	186	0	2	.6	na	108
A very healthy bet.						
Chicken 'n' Vegetable Stir-Fry (Big Boy)	795	109	18	0	na	845
Split this entrée—it's enough for two.						
Chicken Pot Pie (Boston Market)	780	60	47	17	7	930
Skip it. It contains enough fat for an entire day.						
Half a Turkey Carver Sandwich (Boston Market)	390	34	14	4	0	910
A healthy choice.						
Italian Combo Sandwich (Panera Bread)	1100	56	20	0	91	3200
Skip it. It contains more sodium than you should have in an entire day.						
Fried Shrimp Dinner—5 oz (Denny's)	260	18	12	2	0	790
A reasonable choice if you've got to have that crunch.						
Coleslaw—4 oz (Bob Evans)	209	19	14	2	0	242
Stick with raw or cooked vegetables.						
French Fries—2 cups (Steak Escape)	651	87	34	na	na	535
Skip 'em or split them with at least two other people.						
Onion Rings—4 oz (Denny's)	381	38	23	6	0	1003
Skip it. You're just eating breading and fat.						
Baked Potato—plain (Denny's)	220	51	0	0	0	16
A healthy choice.						

Menu Item	Calories	Carbohy-drate (g)	Fat (g)	Saturated Fat (g)	*Trans* Fat (g)	Sodium (mg)
Baked Potato (Loaded with Bacon Bits, Sour Cream, Butter and Cheese)—(Denny's)	506	68	35	20	na	503
Order a baked potato and request one topping to be served on the side. Apply it sparingly.						
Apple Pie—1 slice (Boston Market)	420	56	20	4	5	650
If you must indulge, request at least two forks so you can share it.						

The Menu Profile

Silverware and napkins are generally all that greet you at the tables of lower-priced establishments. When you go more upscale, bread and butter are usually served, and some ethnic eateries offer chips and salsa or breadsticks.

First, you'll be asked if you want appetizers. The crunchy, fried variety are everywhere—and they contain an almost lethal amount of fat and calories. Even healthier choices, such as onions and mushrooms, are battered, dipped, and fried in some of these restaurants; others offer them sautéed. You may also see nachos or super nachos, which are fried tortilla chips with countless high-fat goodies on top—cheese, meat, sour cream, and guacamole. Other tasty appetizers include fried mozzarella sticks, buffalo chicken wings (which are deep-fried and traditionally served with blue cheese dressing), and a battered, deep-fried onion served up with creamy dressing.

There are a few appetizers that can be a healthy portion-controlled main dish, such as shrimp cocktail, peel-and-eat shrimp with cocktail sauce, oysters on the half-shell, a cup of chili, or Mexican pizza. Some appetizer menus also include platters of raw vegetables with creamy dip. The dips are almost always high in fat and calories, but here's menu creativity at work—ask for a side of low-calorie salad dressing instead. If your dining companions order high-fat appetizers, order a healthier appetizer or a garden or spinach salad for yourself. Otherwise it will be hard to resist "tasting" your friends' appetizers.

Soups can go either way—healthy or loaded with fat. Here's a rule of thumb: If you can see through it, or it's loaded with beans and vegetables, it's healthy (but probably also high in sodium). If it's white and/or creamy, it's probably loaded with fat. Most menus include high-fat French onion soup (healthy before cheese and bread are loaded on top, but there's no reason you can't ask them to serve it without them), New England clam chowder, potato soup, or broccoli and cheese soup. Healthier choices include chicken vegetable soup, chicken noodle soup, black bean soup, chili (hold the cheese), and Manhattan clam chowder. If sodium is a concern, it's best to avoid any soup.

Entrées vary tremendously. You'll find salads, sandwiches, burgers with various toppings, filet mignon (a small and relatively lean cut), chicken entrées, fish selections, and other hot meats partnered with a starch and a hot vegetable. Never fear—there are always at least a few healthy choices.

Almost every family-fare menu includes an extensive list of salads. Be sure to pay close attention to what is loaded on top of that healthy bed of greens. House, Cobb, taco, chicken, tuna, Greek, and spinach are the usual choices. Some restaurants serve salads in fried tortilla shells; always request yours in a bowl instead. The shell is just too tempting to have on your plate.

If you choose a salad, look for red and green flag words. Consider the Cobb salad: It includes chicken or turkey breast, bacon, avocado, blue cheese, hard-boiled egg, black olives, and tomatoes—a list that includes both red and green flag words. If you like a salad's basic ingredients, just request that some of the items be left in the kitchen. Replace those ingredients with healthier choices, such as tomatoes, onions, and peppers. Last but not least is the dressing. Dressing can transform a salad from a healthy meal to a nutrition disaster. America's favorites—thousand island and blue cheese—contain at least 70 calories per level tablespoon. Here are a few ways to "dress for success":

- Select reduced-calorie or nonfat dressings.
- Order dressing on the side, so you can control how much you consume.
- Request a side of vinegar or lemon wedges to dilute the dressing.

For more details and nutrition information about salad dressings and suggestions for a healthy approach, read about salads in Chapter 13.

Almost all family-fare menus include plenty of sandwiches. Tuna salad or turkey and ham club sandwiches served on croissants are found on many menus ... and they contain an unbelievable amount of calories and fat. In particular, watch out for healthy-sounding tuna or chicken salads, because they are packed with mayonnaise. Stick with unadulterated meats, like turkey, roast beef, ham, and chicken. Ask the server to hold the mayonnaise and request a side of mustard, low-calorie salad dressing, honey mustard, barbecue sauce, or ketchup instead. If cranberry sauce is on the menu, it makes a delicious and healthy spread for a chicken or turkey sandwich. Mexican hot sauce and horseradish are even lower in calories. Half a sandwich with soup, salad, or a baked potato should make a satisfying meal.

As you consider the sandwiches, carefully check all the ingredients. A healthy grilled chicken breast sandwich might be topped with bacon and cheese. Order sandwiches with healthy preparations—charbroiled, teriyaki, or barbecued—and stick with healthier toppers—sautéed onions, mushrooms and/or peppers, honey mustard, and jalapeño peppers.

Always avoid certain sandwiches, such as Reubens, Philadelphia cheese steaks, clubs, and melts. They ooze with fat—usually because they are loaded with cheese.

Sandwiches are also problematic because they almost always come with potato chips, potato salad, pasta salad, French fries, and/or creamy coleslaw. All of these side items are loaded with fat and calories. Request healthier choices, such as a baked potato, pickle, rice pilaf, green salad, or steamed or sautéed vegetables, instead.

On to one of America's favorite foods—burgers. A family-fare menu without hamburgers with various toppings would be sacrilegious. Meat portions (the quantity of raw meat, that is) on burgers are usually at least 6 ounces and often exceed 10 or 12 ounces. Order a smaller burger ("petite" or "queen" are words that describe smaller meat portions). Also, understand exactly how much meat you'll end up being served. If a menu says its burger features "8 ounces of first-quality ground beef," it usually means that the patty is 8 ounces when it is raw. An 8-ounce raw hamburger will weigh 6 ounces—at most—when it is served because it will lose about 2 ounces during the cooking process. The more well-done it is, the smaller it will be.

You might be avoiding hot entrées because you think salads and sandwiches are lighter and lower in calories. This is a common misconception. Chicken or beef fajitas, a chicken or vegetable stir-fry, or a barbecued chicken breast can be considerably healthier choices, especially if you split them or take half of them home. However, many nutritional disasters lurk in the hot entrée section, including fettuccine Alfredo, barbecued ribs, or high-fat ribeye, T-bone, and porterhouse steaks.

Desserts are best passed by. Cheesecake, flourless chocolate cake, apple pie à la mode, and ice cream sundaes turn up on most menus. Once in a while, you'll see fruit sorbet or frozen yogurt. Decent choices are fruit pies (hold the ice cream or whipped cream), sorbet, and frozen yogurt. If you must eat dessert, remember that portions are huge, so place the order with the understanding that you will share it with your dining companions.

Those Kids' Menus

Family-fare restaurants almost always provide kids' menus, which feature what adults think kids like to eat—fried chicken strips, hamburgers, and hot dogs—all served with fries. Some also offer pizza or pasta with tomato sauce. Read Chapter 6 to learn more about kids' menus—and how to help the kids in your life learn healthy restaurant eating habits.

▷ Green Flag Words

Ingredients

- △ sautéed onions, peppers, mushrooms
- △ jalapeño peppers
- △ barbecue sauce
- △ cocktail sauce
- △ horseradish
- △ mustard, honey mustard
- △ lettuce, sliced tomatoes, raw onions
- △ spicy Mexican beef or chicken
- △ low-calorie or nonfat salad dressing

Cooking Methods/Menu Descriptions/Names

△ marinated in teriyaki sauce
△ Cajun or blackened
△ mesquite-grilled
△ charbroiled or grilled
△ stir-fried
△ marinated
△ barbecued
△ steamed

▶ Red Flag Words

Ingredients

▼ cheese (grated, melted, topped with, smothered in, sauce)
▼ blue cheese (crumbled, topped with, salad dressing)
▼ guacamole
▼ bacon (strips, crumbled, crisp)
▼ sausage
▼ sour cream
▼ butter or cream
▼ mayonnaise, garlic mayonnaise, "special or house" sauce

Cooking Methods/Menu Descriptions/Names

▼ golden fried, crispy fried
▼ deep-fried
▼ lightly fried
▼ battered and fried
▼ rolled in bread crumbs and fried or sautéed
▼ loaded or topped with cheese, bacon, or sour cream
▼ served in or on a crisp tortilla shell
▼ large, jumbo, piled high, stacked
▼ Alfredo

At the Table

- ▼ butter, margarine
- ▼ mayonnaise
- ▼ sour cream

Special Requests

- ♦ "On the blackened chicken sandwich, please leave off the cheese and add sautéed mushrooms and onions?"
- ♦ "On the roast beef sandwich, can you make sure they don't put any butter or mayonnaise on the bread? Instead, I'd like a side of mustard or horseradish."
- ♦ "Do you have Mexican hot sauce or vinegar? Could I get a bit to use on my salad?"
- ♦ "Please hold the sour cream, but you can load on the lettuce and tomato."
- ♦ "Please bring me a little bowl of low-calorie salad dressing that I can use as a vegetable dip."
- ♦ "Can I substitute a baked potato for the French fries?"
- ♦ "Could you leave the fries off the plate and substitute the vegetable of the day?"
- ♦ "Could I get that sandwich on whole-grain bread instead of a croissant?"
- ♦ "We are going to split the salad and the hamburger, so please bring an extra plate."
- ♦ "We are going to split the steak and baked potato. Can we also have a side order of a green vegetable or garden salad?"

Typical Menu: American Style

✷ *Indicates preferred choices*

Appetizers

Nachos (nacho chips covered with melted cheese and jalapeño peppers with a side of salsa)

Super nachos (nacho chips covered with melted Monterey Jack cheese, refried beans, spicy beef or chicken, shredded lettuce and tomatoes, and a side of salsa)

Buffalo chicken wings (lightly fried marinated chicken wings in a hot and spicy sauce, served with blue cheese dressing)

✷ **Peel-and-eat shrimp** (½ lb. of steamed shrimp served with cocktail sauce)

Potato skins (fried potato skins filled with cheese and a choice of bacon bits, sour cream, or onions)

Mozzarella sticks (mozzarella cheese rolled in breadcrumbs and fried; served with marinara sauce)

✷ **Raw bar platter** (oysters on the half-shell, steamed clams, and jumbo shrimp served with cocktail sauce)

Chicken fingers (chicken breast tenders breaded and fried, served with a dipping sauce)

Fried whole onion (a battered and deep-fried onion served with creamy dipping sauce)

Soups (served in a cup or a bowl)

A cup of soup is a great filler, and a bowl of soup can substitute for an entrée.

New England clam chowder (creamy chowder with clams and potatoes, served with oyster crackers)

✷ **French onion soup** (smothered with Swiss cheese). (Note: request holding the cheese and bread and it's OK.)

✿ **Chili** (spicy mixture of pinto beans, ground beef, and sautéed onions and peppers, topped with onions and Monterey Jack cheese)

✿ **Vegetable gumbo** (blend of garden vegetables, onions, tomatoes, broccoli, and green beans simmered in Cajun spices)

✿ **Black bean** (hearty black beans simmered for hours with onions, peppers and cilantro)

Salads

Consider eliminating or limiting such high-fat ingredients as avocado, olives, bacon, cheese, croutons, and and eggs. Ask that the dressing be served on the side.

✿ **Seafood pasta salad** (pasta topped with baby shrimp and bell peppers, tossed with Italian dressing, and served on a bed of mixed greens) (Note: Ask that the Italian dressing be served on the side.)

✿ **Blackened chicken salad** (slices of marinated and blackened chicken breast, mixed salad greens, avocado slices, cherry tomatoes, broccoli, shredded Swiss cheese, and croutons)

✿ **Chef salad** (julienned turkey, ham, and Swiss cheese served on bed of lettuce with diced tomatoes and red and green pepper, all in crispy tortilla shell) (Note: Ask the server to bring the salad in a dish rather than a tortilla shell.)

✿ **House salad** (a blend of greens with sliced cucumbers and tomatoes and alfalfa sprouts)

✿ **Cobb salad** (a bed of greens topped with chicken, avocado, olives, and blue cheese)

✿ **Spinach salad** (fresh spinach topped with sliced mushrooms, eggs, and bacon bits, served with hot bacon dressing)

Salad Dressings

You can always request olive oil and vinegar, a much healthier choice.

House (creamy garlic)
Ranch
❀ **Italian**
❀ **French**
Blue cheese
Thousand island
Hot bacon
❀ **Balsamic vinaigrette**
❀ **Low-calorie ranch**
❀ **Low-calorie Italian**
❀ **Nonfat honey mustard**

Sandwiches

Sandwiches are usually served with French fries and creamy coleslaw. Always ask for lower-calorie side items such as salads, cooked vegetables, or baked potatoes. Also ask the server to hold the cheese or bacon.

❀ **French dip** (thinly sliced beef, melted provolone cheese, and natural gravy)
❀ **Chicken sandwich** (a marinated breast of chicken blackened on the grill and topped with lettuce, tomatoes, and sprouts)
Tuna melt (creamy tuna salad topped with melted Swiss cheese)
Seafood salad croissant (a croissant filled with a mixture of creamy seafood salad, celery, and onions)

Burgers

Burgers are usually served with sliced tomato, lettuce, French fries, and a side of creamy coleslaw. Regular hamburger patties are usually around 6 ounces of ground beef; and jumbo patties range from 9 to 12 ounces. Substitute healthier sides and order the smaller burger unless you are sharing.

✿ **American hamburger**
   Cheeseburger (with a slice of Swiss or Cheddar cheese)
   Bacon cheeseburger (with several slices of bacon and a slice of Monterey Jack cheese)
✿ **Veggie burger** (with sautéed onions, peppers, and mushrooms)
   Chili burger (with spicy Mexican chili)

Hot Entrées

✿ **Fajitas** (a choice of chicken or beef grilled with onions and green peppers and served with warm flour tortillas and sides of sour cream, guacamole, salsa, and Mexican hot sauce)
   Baby back ribs (a robust portion served with fried onion rings and baked beans)
✿ **Teriyaki chicken breast** (served with rice pilaf and sautéed vegetables)
✿ **Filet mignon** (a 7-ounce cut of grilled prime aged beef)
   Chicken-fried steak (a sirloin steak dipped in batter and fried and served with country gravy, a baked potato, and steamed vegetables)
✿ **Oriental stir-fry** (choice of chicken, shrimp, or vegetables served over Chinese egg noodles)
   Prime rib (a pound of boneless prime rib)

Fettuccine Alfredo (wide noodles covered with our creamy and cheesy Alfredo sauce)

Combinations

Always choose a broth- or bean-based soup.

✿ **Soup and salad** (a bowl of any soup and a house salad)
Quiche and salad (a slice of ham, broccoli, and mushroom quiche served with house salad)
✿ **Soup or salad and half sandwich** (soup or a house salad with half a sandwich)

Side Orders

Always ask for butter or sour cream to be served on the side.

French fries
Creamy coleslaw
✿ **Rice pilaf**
✿ **Baked potato** with butter and/or sour cream (Note: The portion size may be big enough to split.)
✿ **Sautéed vegetables**

Desserts

Be sure to ask for plenty of forks.

✿ **Deep-dish apple pie à la mode** (vanilla ice cream) (Note : Hold the ice cream.)
New York cheesecake (topped with choice of strawberry or blueberry sauce)
Ice cream (two scoops of vanilla, chocolate, or strawberry)
Hot fudge sundae
✿ **Sorbet** (two scoops of raspberry or lemon sherbet)

··················· ◀ **"May I Take Your Order?"** ▶ ···················

Low-Calorie Sample Meal

Peel-and-eat shrimp
Quantity: 1 order (9–12 med. shrimp)
Cocktail sauce
Quantity: 2 tablespoons
Oriental stir-fry, vegetable
Quantity: 1½ cups
Chinese egg noodles
Quantity: 1 cup
Sorbet, raspberry
Quantity: ¾ cup (½ order)
Mineral water
Quantity: unlimited

NUTRITION SUMMARY
610 calories
Carb: 88 g, 58%
Fat: 14 g, 21%
Protein: 32 g, 21%
Cholesterol: 227 mg (high because of the shrimp)
Sodium: 970 mg

Moderate-Calorie Sample Meal

House salad (dressing on the side)
Quantity: 2 cups
Blue cheese dressing (ask for vinegar to thin the dressing)
Quantity: 1 tablespoon
Teriyaki chicken breast
Quantity: 4 oz.
Rice pilaf
Quantity: 1 cup
Sautéed vegetables
Quantity: 1 cup
Wine
Quantity: 1 glass (6 oz.)

NUTRITION SUMMARY
760 calories
Carb: 60 g, 32%
Fat: 26 g, 31%
Protein: 42 g, 22%
Alcohol: 115 calories as alcohol (15%)
Cholesterol: 120 mg
Sodium: 1170 mg

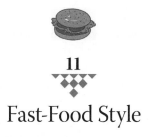

11

Fast-Food Style

Today, fast-food restaurants are a ubiquitous part of our fast-paced, on-the-go culture. As a group, these quick-service restaurants represent the largest segment of restaurants in the U.S., feeding millions of people daily. Fast-food franchises are springing up all over the developing world, and their presence is believed by some to be a significant factor in the worldwide obesity epidemic.

However, it's important to give credit where credit is due. Today, you can use the words "fast food" and "healthy" in the same breath, as restaurants like McDonald's, Burger King, and Wendy's introduce more vegetables and fruits on their menus and offer a few healthy beverages as well. With a little knowledge, effort, and willpower, you can eat a reasonably healthy fast-food meal.

"Fast food" conjures up thoughts of burgers, fries, and soda, but today many other restaurant foods are served up fast. Many fast-food outlets serve pizza, subs, Mexican food, or Chinese food. Some fast-food establishments only serve their food to-go, but most also offer seating areas. This chapter concentrates on what's served in traditional fast-food chains: burgers, fried chicken, chicken sandwiches, roast beef sandwiches, fries, and soda. You'll find information about other foods served fast in the cuisine-specific chapters. *Eat Out, Eat Right* contains information about every food served fast, including pizza, breakfast, sandwich shops, and even ethnic cuisines, such as Mexican and Chinese.

Fast-food restaurants began to line America's highways and byways in the 1950s and 1960s. Their basic menus of burgers, fries, and soda were augmented over the years with new entrée items, breakfast items, and desserts. During the 1980s, fast-food restaurant chains took a few stabs at nutrition consciousness. Most chains introduced leaner burgers, grilled chicken sandwiches, baked potatoes, salads, lower-fat salad dressings, and lowfat milk, but many of the healthier items were eventually dropped from menus because they didn't sell.

The invention of the super-sized burger, fries, and soda combo in the 1990s made fast-food profits and American waistlines expand dramatically. McDonald's voluntarily withdrew its "super size" promotion that encouraged patrons to increase the sizes of their often sugary beverages and French fries for a nominal fee, but in many restaurants mammoth burgers and chicken sandwiches continue to be the norm.

Lately, fast-food outlets have begun to include healthier options. For example, McDonald's now offers a variety of salads with lowfat dressings, apple-walnut salad in two sizes, and fruit and yogurt parfaits. Burger King offers a veggie burger. Wendy's tried a fresh fruit cup that didn't sell, but the chain is back with mandarin oranges and yogurt with granola. Most fast-food chains offer lowfat regular and chocolate milk and apple and orange juice. In kids' meals, McDonald's now offers apple slices with lowfat caramel sauce and Burger King offers applesauce as alternatives to French fries. They are trying to offer good choices, and it's up to consumers to order these foods if they are to remain on the menus.

On occasion, most Americans will find themselves in a fast-food restaurant. Sometimes it's unavoidable. For families with young children, the drive-through window can be a necessary evil. Fast-food meals are quick, dependable, accessible, and relatively inexpensive. In fact, there are actually a few pluses to fast-food restaurants to help you eat healthy—no foods greet you when you sit down at the table, and you can choose the portions you want. Read on to learn how to apply Chapter 4's skills and strategies for healthier eating when you eat fast food.

Nutrition Snapshot

The following nutrition snapshot is intended to provide you with the nutrition numbers for many common menu items served at fast-food restaurants covered in this chapter. Today, most large fast-food chains provide extensive nutrition information in two forms: online on their websites and in brochures or boards posted in the restaurants.

If you choose to check out fast-food nutrition information on the restaurant's website, look for a link that clearly indicates that it leads to nutrition information, or simply type "nutrition" into the site's search engine. Most of the chains provide their nutrition information in a downloadable and printable PDF file, and some also enable you to put together an order, leaving out or putting in various sandwich toppers and other side items to calculate a complete and accurate estimate of the nutrition facts for the entire meal that you will eat.

In the chart below, you'll see nutrition data that ranges from mind-blowing to healthy. Use them to learn about the nutrition profiles of your current favorite fast-food meals. If necessary, change your favorites to healthier alternatives. As you will see in the chart Little Changes Make a Big Difference on page 104, you can have a healthy and delicious meal at most fast-food restaurants. Because the extensiveness of the exact nutrition information provided in the nutrition snapshot chart, there is no typical menu in this chapter.

Menu Item	Calories	Carbohydrate (g)	Fat (g)	Saturated Fat (g)	*Trans* Fat (g)	Sodium (mg)
Single Hamburgers						
Hamburger (BK)	290	30	12	5	0	560
Cheeseburger (MD)	300	33	12	6	.5	750
Homestyle Hamburger (DQ)	290	29	12	5	0	630
Single Classic with Everything (W)	430	37	20	7	1	900
Jr. Hamburger (W)	280	34	9	3.5	.5	590

Stick with a single-patty, regular, or junior burger or cheeseburger. There is no need to pile on toppings or sauces.

Deluxe Hamburgers						
Quarter-Pounder with Cheese (MD)	510	40	26	12	1.5	1190
Big Mac (MD)	540	45	29	10	1.5	1040
Whopper with Cheese (BK)	760	52	47	13	1.5	880
Bacon Double Cheeseburger (BK)	360	31	18	8	.5	870
Monster Thickburger (H)	1420	46	108	43	na	2770

Skip 'em.

Roast Beef Sandwiches						
Junior Roast Beef (A)	272	34	10	4	0	740
Regular Roast Beef (A)	320	34	14	5	.5	953
Super Roast Beef (A)	398	40	19	6	.5	1060
Roast Beef and Swiss (A)	777	73	41	13	1.5	1743

The smaller they are, the healthier they are.

Grilled Chicken Sandwiches						
Tendergrill—No Sauce or Mayo (BK)	400	49	7	1.5	0	1090
Tendergrill—with Mayo (BK)	510	49	19	3.5	.5	1180
Premium Grilled Chicken Classic (MD)	420	51	10	2	0	1190
Chargrilled Chicken Sandwich (CF)	270	33	3.5	1	0	940
Chargrilled chicken club sandwich (CF)	380	33	11	5	0	1240

A healthier bet, particularly when you hold the mayo and the special sauce. Opt for a lower-fat sauce, such as barbecue or honey mustard.

Menu Item	Calories	Carbohy-drate (g)	Fat (g)	Saturated Fat (g)	*Trans* Fat (g)	Sodium (mg)
Fried Chicken Sandwiches						
Spicy Chicken Fillet Sandwich (W)	440	46	16	3	0	1320
McChicken—(MD)	360	40	16	3.5	1	790
Premium Crispy Chicken Club Sandwich (MD)	570	52	21	7	0	1720
Chick 'n' Crisp Sandwich (BK)	480	36	31	5	2	870
Big Chicken Fillet Sandwich (H)	800	76	37	6	na	1890
Chick-Fil-A Chicken Sandwich (CF)	410	38	16	3.5	0	1300
Opt for grilled.						
Chicken Pieces						
Chicken Tenders—6 pieces (BK)	250	16	15	3.5	2.5	720
Chicken McNuggets—6 pieces (MD)	250	15	15	3	1.5	670
Chicken Nuggets—5 pieces (W)	230	12	15	3	0	520
Crispy Strips—3 pieces (KFC)	350	16	19	3.5	0	1190
Skip this and opt for grilled chicken or a single burger.						
Sauces for Chicken Pieces						
Honey Mustard—2 Tbsp. (BK)	90	8	6	1	0	180
Barbecue—2 Tbsp. (W)	45	10	0	0	0	170
Honey Mustard—2 Tbsp. (MD)	50	12	0	0	0	0
Sweet 'n' Sour—2 Tbsp. (MD)	50	12	0	0	0	150

Use the lower-calorie and fat choices as a substitute for the typical mayonnaise based sauces used on sandwiches.

Menu Item	Calories	Carbohydrate (g)	Fat (g)	Saturated Fat (g)	*Trans* Fat (g)	Sodium (mg)
Fried Chicken Pieces						
Original Breast—1 piece (KFC)	360	7	21	5	0	1020
Original Drumstick—1 piece (KFC)	130	2	8	2	0	350
Extra Crispy Breast—1 piece (KFC)	440	15	27	6	0	970
Extra Crispy Drumstick (KFC)	160	6	10	2	0	370
Original Thigh—1 piece (CC)	330	8	23	6	3	680
Spicy wing—1 piece (CC)	300	7	19	5	3	540

Skip 'em unless you've just got to have a piece or two; if so, stick with a breast or drumstick and peel off the skin before eating.

Fried Fish Sandwiches						
Big Fish Sandwich (BK)	640	67	32	6	2.5	1450
Filet-o-Fish (MD)	380	38	18	4	1	660

Skip 'em. They are a nutrition disaster.

French Fries (salted)						
Small (MD)	250	30	13	2.5	305	140
Medium (MD)	380	47	20	4	5	220
Small (BK)	230	26	13	3	3	380
Medium (BK)	360	41	13	3	3	590
Small (W)	330	42	16	2.5	.5	340
Large (W)	520	69	24	3.5	1	550

Eat only a small amount. Order a small size or split a large one.

Baked Potatoes						
Plain (W)	270	61	0	0	0	25
With Sour Cream and Chives (W)	320	63	4	2.5	0	55

A healthy option, but watch what gets added on top. At Wendy's, a baked potato and a small cup of chili can make a delicious, healthy meal.

Menu Item	Calories	Carbohy-drate (g)	Fat (g)	Saturated Fat (g)	*Trans* Fat (g)	Sodium (mg)
Milkshakes						
Vanilla—small (BK)	400	57	15	9	0	240
Chocolate—king (BK)	1260	204	38	24	1	640
Chocolate Triple Thick—small (MD)	440	76	10	6	.5	190
Vanilla Frosty—small (W)	310	52	8	5	0	180
Vanilla Frosty Float with Coca-Cola (W)	410	78	8	5	0	190
Jamocha—large (A)	647	107	17	10	.5	509
Avoid or split 'em.						
Desserts						
Cookies—1 pkg. (MD)	270	39	11	6	0	170
Fruit 'n' Yogurt Parfait (MD)	160	31	2	1	0	85
Baked Apple Pie (MD)	270	36	12	3.5	5	190
Cherry Turnover (A)	377	65	15	5	6	201
Peanut Butter Parfait (DQ)	730	99	31	17	0	180
Cheesecake—1 slice (CF)	340	30	21	12	1	270
Fudge Nut Brownie—1 piece (CF)	330	45	15	3.5	2.5	210
Skip 'em. They're simply not worth the calories.						

Abbreviations:

A: Arby's
BK: Burger King
CC: Church's Chicken
CF: Chick-fil-A
DQ: Dairy Queen

H: Hardee's
JB: Jack in the Box
KFC: KFC
MD: McDonalds
W: Wendy's

Little Changes Make a Big Difference

In the "Little Changes Make a Big Difference" chart, you'll see how small changes in an order add up to a big nutrition difference in fast-food restaurants. Changes in the size of an order, its preparation, or its accompanying beverage can easily help you create a healthier fast-food meal.

Food Choice	Calories	Fat (g) (unsaturated)	Sodium (mg)
Change This Order:			
Quarter-Pound Hamburger with Cheese and Sauces	510	26	1190
French Fries (large)	570	30	330
Regular Soda (12 oz.)	140	0	6
Totals	**1220**	**56**	**1526**
To:			
Hamburger (Single without Cheese)	250	9	520
French Fries (½ a medium order)	190	10	110
Diet Soda (12 oz.)	1	0	30
Totals	**441**	**19**	**660**
Change This Order:			
Fried Chicken Sandwich	570	25	1145
French Fries (large)	520	27	685
Lowfat Chocolate Shake, (small)	385	9	170
Totals	**1475**	**61**	**2000**
To:			
Grilled Chicken Sandwich with No Mayo and 1 Tbsp. Barbecue Sauce	385	6	850
French Fries, Large (½ order)	285	15	165
Diet Soda (12 oz.)	1	0	30
Totals	**671**	**21**	**1045**

The Menu Profile

The bitter truth is this: Most items on fast-food menus are high in total fat, saturated fat, and sodium, and are low in healthier carbohydrates. Even a nutritious food like a potato is usually drenched in from the oil of the deep-fryer or smothered by lots of unhealthy cheese, bacon, and sour cream. There's not much that is green and crunchy in an order of burger, fries, and a shake.

You should minimize the amount of fried foods you eat for several reasons. Firstly, cutting down on total fat will decrease the amount of calories you consume. Also, many fried foods contain *trans* fats (learn more about *trans* fats and how to avoid them in Chapter 2), which are unhealthy. If you must indulge in some fried food, offset it with a grilled or nonfried item. For example, opt for a small order of French fries (or share a medium order) with a no-frills hamburger, a grilled chicken sandwich, or a roast beef sandwich. If you choose a piece or two of fried chicken, remove the skin before you eat it and add a plain baked potato, a garden salad, and baked beans or an ear of corn.

Fat grams add up in other parts of the meal as well. Think about the toppings on those main dishes: cheese, bacon, and "special sauces"—which are usually either mayonnaise-based or just plain mayonnaise. All are loaded with fat and contain at least some unhealthy saturated fat.

Even healthier options like salads and baked potatoes usually have significant amounts of fat tucked away in their dressings and toppings. Consider the fast food packets of salad dressing: Many contain as much as four tablespoons of dressing and more than 200 calories. If you pour on the whole packet, you destroy the health benefits of the salad. The same logic holds true for the nonfat baked potato offered at some fast-food franchises. When you add cheese sauces, sour cream, and/or bacon bits, you're pouring on fat. But that's one of the great things about fast food: You are in control. You can specify exactly how you want your food "dressed."

The high sodium content of fast-food meals is another pitfall. Sodium levels shoot through the roof as foods are coated in salty batters and served with pickles, sauces, bacon, cheese, and salad dressing. Of course, you can't mention sodium and fast food without considering the amount of salt in French fries. Remember—you can order them salt-free.

Entrées are loaded with salt, too. Burger King's Original Whopper with cheese contains more than 1,400 milligrams of sodium—more than half the maximum daily amount for adults. In fact, it is commonplace for fast-food meals to rise above the desirable daily sodium count of 2,300 milligrams. Some of the sodium is difficult to cut out because of the high sodium content of the packaged foods the restaurants use. A chicken fillet contains around 600 milligrams of sodium before it even hits the deep fryer. Cut your sodium intake where you can by cutting down on high-sodium ingredients like salad dressing, cheese, sauces, and bacon. You'll be cutting back the fat as well.

Surprisingly, the art of preplanning is actually easier in fast-food restaurants. You probably know the menu intimately before you even set foot in the restaurant. Decide what you'll order before you cross the threshold or shout your order into the drive-thru speaker. Once you are in the restaurant, the smells and visual cues might tempt you to change your mind, but hold firm. If you are dining with a companion, give her or him your order before you walk in and head to the dining room to secure a table.

Another advantage of fast-food restaurants is that you don't have to wait to eat. You'll be eating as soon as you sit down. There's no bread and butter on the table or high-fat appetizers.

Dessert is rarely a temptation. Portion size is easy to control as long as you order foods with the words small, regular, junior, or single. Avoid any of the words that are fast-food-speak for large portions: giant, super, jumbo, double, triple, big, and extra large. A single hamburger has between two and three ounces of meat, which is just about the right portion for lunch or dinner.

Although you've probably chosen a fast-food restaurant because you're short on time, you should monitor your pace of eating. Take at least 15 to 20 minutes to consume your meal. Avoid the drive-thru if you can. If you are eating in the car, you can't focus on the food. You'll hardly taste it as you shovel it in.

Hamburgers

Unfortunately, the trend in fast-food hamburgers is bigger is better. Most fast-food burger chains offer double, triple, quad (4 patties), biggie, or monster burgers. Most of these are also loaded with high-fat toppings, such as cheese, bacon, and special sauce. Vegetables are scarce. Avoid these giant burgers and order small ones instead.

The frequent additions of cheese, special sauces (usually mayonnaise-based), and bacon add fat and calorie, but pickles, onions, lettuce, tomatoes, mustard, and ketchup increase flavor without the fat. Compare the difference between a plain hamburger at Burger King, with about 300 calories and 12 grams of fat (40 percent of calories), to their Double Whopper with Cheese, with about 600 calories and 35 grams of fat (50 percent of calories).

Roast Beef Sandwiches

Arby's is famous for its roast beef sandwiches, and several other chains have added beef sandwiches to their growing list of menu items. Arby's regular or junior roast beef sandwich without cheese is in the vicinity of the 30 percent fat goal and could be a better choice than a hamburger. As with the burgers, avoid the high-fat extras—cheese, melted cheese, creamy dressings and sauces (for example, Arby's Horsey Sauce contains 5 grams of fat and about 60 calories per tablespoon). Feel free to use spicy barbecue sauce, honey mustard, mustard, or unadulterated horseradish for extra punch.

Chicken Sandwiches

Today, most of the chains whose roots were in burgers and fries now also serve at least one grilled and one fried chicken sandwich. KFC, the chicken king among restaurant chains, serves three reasonably healthy chicken sandwiches—Tender Roast, Honey BBQ and Oven Roasted Twister. Any of them are healthier (lower in fat) if you skip the sandwiches' special sauce. Chick-Fil-A, which is not as commonplace as KFC, also offers healthier chicken options, including chargrilled chicken sandwiches and wraps. McDonald's and Burger King also offer grilled chicken sandwiches.

If you ask the cashier to hold the sauce, a grilled chicken sandwich is healthier than a loaded hamburger, fried chicken sandwich, or fried chicken pieces, such as nuggets or tenders. Always look for the word grilled in the description: If you don't see it, you can bet that the chicken is fried. Today, most restaurants that serve a grilled chicken sandwich also offer fried chicken pieces with lowfat sauces like barbecue or honey mustard. Request some of this sauce for your grilled chicken sandwich (they're tasty on burgers, too).

Chicken Pieces (Nuggets or Tenders)

Fried chicken pieces were first introduced by McDonald's and are now offered by most chains. They are a hit with kids because they are easy to eat, but they are coated, deep-fried, and loaded with fat—about 50 percent of their calories come from fat. (A few chains, such as Chick-Fil-A, do offer these grilled, which is a healthy choice.) There are too many healthy alternatives to even consider eating these.

Fried Chicken

A few chains specialize in serving fried chicken. Several of them tried doing roast chicken, but it didn't last. Kentucky Fried Chicken, or KFC, as it now wants to be called to avoid the "F" word, is the leader in the field. There's little nutritional value in fried chicken. If you eat fried chicken once in a blue moon, eat no more than one or two pieces and always choose the breast. Save fat and calories by removing the skin before eating the chicken, and complement it with healthier sides: mashed potatoes, corn on the cob, green beans, or baked beans.

Fried Fish Sandwiches

Fish is healthy, of course, but not when it's drowned in batter, oil, tartar sauce, and cheese. Fast-food fried fish sandwiches are probably one of the least healthy choices on the menu. These sandwiches average nearly 500 calories and 50 percent fat. Unfortunately, fast-food outlets just don't offer grilled fish. Skip the fish when you're eating fast food; instead, make it at home or order it grilled or broiled in a sit-down restaurant.

French Fries

It seems that nearly every fast-food sandwich is accompanied by crispy golden French fries. They are very hard to pass up, especially once you enter the restaurant and smell them. A small or regular order of French fries isn't horrible—200 to 300 calories. Potatoes are a vegetable and offer some nutritional value.

Unfortunately, they often also contain *trans* fat because of the hydrogenated shortenings in which they are often cooked. If you must have them, share them with a dining companion. Always order a small size and order them salt-free if you want to save a few hundred milligrams of sodium.

Baked Potatoes

Baked potatoes appear on some fast-food menus, but Wendy's is the only national burger chain that has consistently offered them for years. Potatoes are inherently healthy, but avoid loading on fat-containing toppers like butter, margarine, cheese, bacon, and sour cream. Instead, choose lighter toppings like broccoli or chili, without the cheese. Wendy's value menu offers a plain baked potato and a small chili. If you leave off the sour cream, you can have a delicious, filling, low-calorie, and healthy meal. Another option is to split a baked potato in lieu of fries with a dining companion.

Salads

A wide variety of salads—side, garden, chicken, chef, and more—are available at most national burger, roast beef, and chicken chains. Clearly, a side or garden salad with a sandwich is a far healthier alternative to French fries. Better yet, opt for a meal-size salad at Wendy's or Chick-Fil-A, but skip the high-fat add-ons—sour cream, Chinese noodles, nuts, and the like. You must also use the ridiculously large servings of salad dressing sparingly. Choose a lowfat or nonfat salad dressing if you like the taste, but even these should be used judiciously. They might not have the calories, but their sodium count can be sky high. If you like a regular dressing best, make sure you leave more in the packet than you put on your relatively small salad.

Shakes

The shakes pack a lot of calories from carbohydrates, most of which are sugars. Surprisingly, however, some of them are fairly low in fat. The servings are large. Treat them as you would ice cream or other dessert. Order a small shake as an occasional dessert to satisfy your sweet tooth. Request an extra cup and split it.

Desserts

Desserts are easy to avoid in fast-food restaurants. For the most part, they aren't very good, and since a server doesn't come around after the meal to tempt you with them, they are rarely a factor. If you must indulge, order a small ice cream, a frozen yogurt, or an order of cookies. Share the dessert if you are able. Skip the pies, sundaes, and cheesecakes and save your calories for something tastier.

Beverages

By far, the best beverage picks are water and lowfat or nonfat milk. Sometimes fruit juices, usually apple or orange, are available. Avoid the sugar-loaded lemonade and fruit punch, unless a diet alternative is offered. They contain calories with no nutrition and are no better than any other regular soft drink. Any noncaloric diet soft drinks, unsweetened iced tea, or hot coffee or tea without sugar or milk are good alternatives. Check out Chapter 7 for a complete review of nonalcoholic beverages.

···················· ◆ **"May I Take Your Order"** ◆ ··················

Low-Calorie Sample Meal

Baked potato with chili and
cheese
Quantity: 1
**Low-calorie carbonated
beverage**
Quantity: unlimited

> **NUTRITION SUMMARY**
> 480 calories
> Carb: 55 g, 46%
> Fat: 19 g, 35%
> Protein: 23 g, 19%
> Cholesterol: 31 mg
> Sodium: 701 mg

Low-Calorie Sample Meal

Grilled chicken sandwich
with lettuce, tomatoes, and
other vegetables. (Note: Ask
them to hold the special
sauce and use a small amount
of barbecue sauce or honey
mustard.)
Quantity: 1
Garden salad
Quantity: regular size
Reduced-calorie Italian dressing
Quantity: 2 tbsp.
Lowfat milk
Quantity: 8 oz.

> **NUTRITION SUMMARY**
> 495 calories
> Carb: 58 g, 47% fat
> Fat: 14 g, 25%
> Protein: 35 g, 28%
> Cholesterol: 48 mg
> Sodium: 1180 mg

Moderate-Calorie Sample Meal

Hamburger (no cheese)
Quantity: 1
French fries
Quantity: small order
Side salad
Quantity: 1
Reduced-calorie ranch dressing
Quantity: 1 tbsp.
Low-calorie carbonated beverage
Quantity: medium

NUTRITION SUMMARY
620 calories
Carb: 65 g, 42%
Fat: 30 g, 42%
Protein: 25 g, 16%
Cholesterol: 80 mg
Sodium: 870 mg

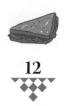

12

Soup 'n' Sandwich Style

In the past, foods like soup, sandwiches, subs, and entrée salads were considered lunch items. They are still popular lunch choices, but many people also choose them for dinner. Americans love sandwiches, more today than ever before, mostly because they are excellent meals for multitasking. Because sandwiches don't require cutlery, harried folks can also drive a car and/or read e-mails while chowing down (but I don't recommend doing so, particularly the driving part!). Wrap-style sandwiches have exploded in popularity, at least partially because they can be eaten with only one hand. Although you might think of a soup and sandwich as a lighter meal, if you don't order with care, these meals can contain just as many calories and just as much fat and sodium as a hot meal at a family-fare restaurant.

The chain restaurants in which you can grab soup, a wrap or sandwich, or an entrée salad have multiplied over the last decade. Au Bon Pain, Panera Bread, Atlanta Bread Company, and Schlotzsky's Deli are established chains in this genre. They all offer menus that focus on soups, fresh breads, and sandwiches.

Sub shops are everywhere. One great feature: Most don't offer fries, so you're not tempted by them. The most popular chains are Subway, Blimpie Subs and Salads, and Quiznos, which differentiates its line by stressing its hot sandwiches (Subway has responded by introducing extensive lines of hot sandwiches as well). These restaurants serve narrow menus centered on sub sandwiches, wraps, and salads. Many smaller chains are also expanding, such as Potbelly Sandwich Works, Charley's Grilled Subs, Rising Roll, Frootz, and Great Wraps. These are just a few of the names you are likely to see in your neighborhood soon, depending on what region of the country you live in. Arby's is also included in this chapter (information about some of their food can be found in Chapter 11: Fast-Food Style as well) because of its extensive sandwich offerings. In addition to their locations in metropolitan areas and suburban strip malls, you'll find sandwich shops in airports, train stations, hospitals, universities, and food courts everywhere.

Do you find yourself on automatic pilot at sandwich shops? Do you order the same tuna or chicken salad sandwich or Italian cold-cut sub with a bag of chips every time? And do you down a 20-ounce soda while you're at it? Catch a glimpse of the nutrition facts for one of these common orders:

A 6-inch tuna salad sandwich served on whole-wheat bread and topped with lettuce and tomato is about 500 calories. Add a bag of potato chips and you'll add another 200 calories. A 20-ounce container of regular soda adds yet another 250 calories. You may not think you're having a big meal, but suddenly you've consumed almost 1,000 calories. And then there's yummy-looking giant cookies right next to the register ... another 300 to 400 calories.

Such a meal doesn't contain that much food, but it contains hundreds of calories from fat and sugar. The good news is that it is easy to eat healthier in soup and sandwich shops. Most sub shops offer small subs. Many of them also offer soup and a half-sandwich or salad combo meals that keep a lid on portion sizes and calories. A few easy changes can have you ordering healthier in no time. If you frequent these restaurants regularly, this can make a big difference in your eating habits.

Nutrition Snapshot

The following nutrition snapshot is intended to provide you with nutrition data for a handful of common menu items served at soup 'n' sandwich and sub shops. You'll see nutrition data that ranges from mind-blowing to healthy. Use them to educate yourself about the nutrition facts of your current favorite meals in these restaurants. If necessary, make healthier choices. Check out the nutrition snapshot in Chapter 13: Salad Style—Bar, Entrée or Side, as soup 'n' sandwich restaurants commonly offer entrée and side salads. Also consult The Lowdown on Salad Dressings chart on page 134 for more information.

Menu Item	Calories	Carbohydrate (g)	Fat (g)	Saturated Fat (g)	*Trans* Fat (g)	Sodium (mg)
Sandwiches						
Sandwich: Market Fresh Roast Ham and Swiss (Arby's)	705	75	31	8	.5	2103
This is a very large sandwich and the calories reflect that. The mayo is a killer too.						
Sandwich: Ham and Swiss Melt (Arby's)	275	35	6	2	0	1118
A more reasonable choice, even with the cheese.						
Sandwich: Portabella and Mozzarella (Panera Bread)	740	80	35	14	1	1200
High in calories and fat, but it's an OK choice if you split it.						
Sandwich: Sierra Turkey (Panera Bread)	960	80	53	13	.5	2310
It sounds healthy, but the fat creeps in with a chipotle mayo and the asiago cheese bread. On top of that, the sandwich is enormous. Move on to another menu item.						

Menu Item	Calories	Carbohydrate (g)	Fat (g)	Saturated Fat (g)	*Trans* Fat (g)	Sodium (mg)
Sandwich: Mediterranean Veggie (half portion) (Panera Bread)	300	50	6	1.5	0	730
A reasonably healthy choice.						
Sub: Tuna Salad—6-inch (Blimpies)	570	51	32	5	na	790
Choose a different filling that's not loaded with mayonnaise.						
Sub: Roast Beef—6-inch (Blimpies)	340	47	5	1	na	870
A healthy choice.						
Sub: Turkey Breast and Ham— 6-inch (Subway)	290	47	5	1.5	0	1210
A healthy choice other than the sodium count.						
Sandwich: Sierra Smoked Turkey with Raspberry Chipotle Sauce (Quiznos)	350	53	6	0	na	1140
A healthy choice, except for the high amount of sodium.						
Sandwich: Vegetarian—small (Schlotzsky's)	355	52	10	na	0	772
A healthy choice.						
Sandwich: Honey Bourbon Chicken (Quiznos)	359	45	6	1	na	1494
A healthy choice, except for the high amount of sodium.						
Sub: 6" Tuna (Subway)	530	44	31	7	.5	1010
Choose a different filling that's not loaded with mayonnaise.						
Sandwich: Albuquerque Turkey— medium (Schlotzsky's)	964	80	40	na	1	2838
Choose a healthier menu item.						
Sandwich: Turkey and Guacamole— small (Schlotzsky's)	364	54	12	na	0	1300
A healthy choice other than the sodium count.						
Sandwich: Hummus—regular (ToGo's Eatery)	790	104	31	5	na	1710
That healthy-sounding hummus racks up the sodium and has plenty of fat, too. Plenty to split.						

Menu Item	Calories	Carbohy- drate (g)	Fat (g)	Saturated Fat (g)	*Trans* Fat (g)	Sodium (mg)
Sandwich: Corned Beef—medium (Schlotzsky's)	582	77	13	na	0	2350
Calories and fat aren't bad, but it's enough sodium for the whole day.						
Sandwich: Corned Beef Reuben— small (Schlotzsky's)	629	54	28	na	1	1353
Not bad if you've got to have a Reuben. Not great either.						
Soups						
Soup: Vegetarian black bean— 8 oz. (Panera Bread)	160	311	1	0	0	820
A healthy high-fiber choice.						
Soup: Vegetable with Chicken and Rice—8 oz. (Panera Bread)	200	17	10	3	0	700
Combine soup with salad for a healthy meal.						
Soup: Mushroom Trio and Roasted Tomato—8 oz. (Panera Bread)	120	11	8	5	0	610
You'd think the fat content would be high, but it's not. It pays to look at the nutrition facts.						
Salads						
Salad: Greek (Panera Bread)	520	17	48	10	0	1560
Move onto another salad, or ask that the dressing be served on the side.						
Salad: Roadhouse Beef (Blimpies)	225	12	10	6	na	650
A healthy choice.						
Salad: Strawberry Poppyseed (Panera Bread)	200	33	3	0	0	240
A healthy choice.						
Salad: Oven-Roasted Chicken (Subway)	140	11	3	.5	0	400
A healthy choice.						
Salad: Tomato and Fresh Mozzarella (Panera Bread)	720	58	43	20	1.5	950
Split this one and hold or go light on the mozzarella.						

Menu Item	Calories	Carbohy-drate (g)	Fat (g)	Saturated Fat (g)	*Trans* Fat (g)	Sodium (mg)
Smoothies						
Banana Berry Smoothie—original (Jamba Juice)	450	106	1	0	0	105
A must-split.						
Peanut Butter Moo'd—original (Jamba Juice)	840	139	21	4.5	na	480
High in calories and fat. Skip it.						

The Menu Profile

The following are a few general tips to put healthy-eating skills and strategies to work. First, have an action plan. Know what you'll order before you set foot in the restaurant. More often than not, you've been at the restaurant before and know the menu well. Practice menu creativity in sandwich or sub shops, at mall food courts, and in your employee cafeteria. Don't be bashful—specify exactly what ingredients you want and what you don't want.

In many situations where you choose a soup 'n' sandwich or sub meal, you'll be consuming your food in an open seating area or back at the office. Because fruits and vegetables are not easy to find at these restaurants, consider bringing along a portion of ready-to-eat raw vegetables from home, such as baby carrots, grape or cherry tomatoes, celery sticks, or broccoli florets. Bringing a piece of fruit is easy too.

As always, portion control is critical. Choose carefully to keep portions small, and give sharing a chance. Perhaps your dining companion could order a sliced meat sandwich and you order a Greek or large garden salad with dressing on the side. If you share the complementary dishes, you both end up with the perfect balance of vegetables, starches, and protein (meat). Another smart move is the combo meal that offers soup or salad and a half-sandwich.

Last, be assertive. Don't let friends or coworkers drag you to a restaurant with few healthy choices.

For each of the types of restaurants in the soup 'n' sandwich category, you'll find a menu profile and a rundown of healthy, tolerable, and worst choices.

Sandwich Shops

The menus are quite predictable: sandwiches on a variety of breads and rolls, wraps, soups, salads (side or main-course), and a few desserts, like cookies, brownies, or carrot cake. Most restaurants offer a variety of mustards—Dijon, brown, or yellow—and mayonnaise as spreads, and some also feature fancier spreads, like honey mustard, cranberry or chipotle mayonnaise, or chopped onions and olives. There are usually quite a few salad dressing choices that range from healthier lowfat or nonfat types to creamy high-fat varieties.

Healthy Choices

Healthy choices are plentiful. Don't skip all sandwiches simply because you think the breads or rolls are loaded with calories—but remember that large rolls or footlong sandwich breads contain far too much carbohydrate for one person. Sandwiches on focaccia are often large, for example.

In general, however, it's what's between the bread that really matters, so don't just take off the top piece of bread and eat the insides to save calories. Choose a healthy whole-grain bread or opt for a whole grain wrap. As always, skip the croissants—they are loaded with fat.

The best sandwich meats are regular or smoked turkey

breast; roasted, grilled, or barbecued chicken breast; roast beef; and ham. Make sure that the serving size is small—no more than 3 ounces of meat. If there's too much, remove some of the meat or share it with someone else. Be careful with vegetarian sandwiches: Some of them are drenched in fat from salad dressing or cheese.

Sandwiches are usually made to order, often right in front of you. Feel free to make special requests—"Go light on the meat and heavy on the vegetables;" "No, cheese, please;" "Please, no mayonnaise or oil on the sandwich;" and so on. If the shop offers them, use mustard, vinegar, ketchup, barbecue sauce, or lowfat salad dressing to moisten your bread and spice up your sandwich. If it's offered, order a half-sandwich with a cup of healthy soup or a side salad. If not, ask a dining companion to split a sandwich and a bowl of soup or main course salad.

If you've got soup in mind, look for broth-based choices, such as chicken, beef, vegetable with noodles or rice; split pea; lentil; barley; or tomato. A cup of chili is always a healthy choice. Freshly prepared soups are best because they have less sodium than canned ones. Avoid creamy soups, like New England clam chowder, creamy broccoli, and cream of anything.

Tolerable Choices

Most sandwich shops offer healthy-sounding choices like tuna, seafood, crabmeat, or chicken salad. Although seafood and poultry are usually leaner than beef and pork, these salads are made with lots and lots of mayonnaise, and only rarely will you encounter a sandwich-shop mayo-based salad that's made with light or nonfat mayonnaise. Thus these salad spreads, served either in a sandwich or on a salad, aren't nearly as healthy as plain sliced meats. If you must indulge, get it at a restaurant that uses minimal mayonnaise and always ask that no extra mayonnaise be placed on the bread of your sandwich. If the filling is piled too high, take some off or share with a dining companion.

Worst Choices

Sandwich shops offer plenty of unhealthy choices. Avoid egg salad, cheeseburgers or burgers loaded with high-fat items, cheese steak sandwiches, grilled cheese, pimiento cheese, ham salad, and hot dogs. Watch out as well for the melts. It is always best to hold the cheese on any sandwich option. Also steer clear of combination or double-meat sandwiches, which end up with about 6 or more ounces of meat—more protein than you need for the entire day. Club sandwiches should be skipped: They are loaded with bread, bacon, and mayonnaise, and usually cheese as well.

Delicatessens

Although the word "kosher" is often associated with delis, very few kosher delicatessens still exist. Perhaps the word "deli" makes you think of hot pastrami or corned beef piled high on rye or a Kaiser roll, knockwurst on a hot-dog roll, chopped liver, or bagels spread thick with cream cheese and topped with lox (smoked salmon). Most of these foods are high in fat and sodium.

Most delis are independent restaurants, but a few chains do exist, such as Schlotzsky's, Jason's Deli, and McAlister's Deli. Schlotzsky's offers small sandwiches, and McAlister's only uses light mayonnaise. Jason's has a "Slimwiches" menu that lists detailed nutrition information right next to the menu items.

It can be harder to find healthy choices in a deli, but you can find some acceptable foods. Practice portion control from the get-go: Mix and match appetizers, soups, salads, and half-sandwiches.

Healthy Choices

Turkey breast, smoked turkey, lean roast beef, or beef brisket are all healthy choices for simple meat sandwiches. In many delis you can order extra-lean corned beef for an extra charge. At delis, the mountain of meat between the bread is usually a huge concern. It's often difficult to balance the bread or roll atop the giant pile of meat. Carve down the meat by splitting a sandwich and ordering an extra roll or slices of bread; you can easily make two sandwiches out of the meat in one or take off some layers of meat and pack it away in a take-home bag. Try a healthy appetizer as a main course, such as stuffed cabbage or gefilte fish. A fresh-fruit platter with cottage cheese can be a healthy choice, but the portions are usually so large that you can easily split one with a dining companion.

Most chains offer at least a few healthy soup choices, like beet borscht, matzo ball chicken soup, or bean and barley soup. Healthy side orders include a bowl of soup and a roll, crackers, salad, vinegar-based coleslaw, pickled tomatoes, sauerkraut (be careful—it's high in sodium), or marinated vegetables.

Tolerable Choices

Most salad platters can be reasonably healthy choices. Stick with chef, turkey, or grilled chicken salad platters. Skip the mayo-based chicken or tuna salad platters, and if the platters include a creamy macaroni or potato salad, ask the server to substitute tomatoes, carrots, cucumbers, or other healthy side items instead. Always ask for salad dressing on the side. A bagel with cream cheese or veggie cream cheese is OK, but specify that it should be served on the side and spread it lightly (also ask if they offer a light cream cheese—many restaurants do!). Order low-calorie sliced tomatoes and Bermuda (red) onions to top the bagel, and enjoy a cup of soup with it.

Worst Choices

Many unhealthy choices lurk in the columns of a deli's menu. Avoid high-fat cured meats like regular corned beef, hot pastrami, beef bologna, salami, knockwurst, hot dog, liverwurst, and tongue. Also steer clear of combination sandwiches that have 6 ounces or more of meat unless you plan to share your sandwich with more than one other other person.

In particular, Reuben sandwiches are a fat and sodium nightmare. The bread is usually grilled with butter, and the sandwich contains corned beef, melted cheese, thousand island dressing, and coleslaw or sauerkraut. Steer clear.

Sub Shops

Depending on what part of the country you are in, long sandwiches filled with anything from Italian meats to tuna fish are called subs, hoagies, heroes, or grinders. There are independent sub shops in every town. Blimpie and Subway, the leading chains, provide extensive nutrition information for most of their menu items. Quizno's offers similar sandwiches but has positioned itself as a bit more upscale. Quizno's has also chosen to keep its nutrition data a secret, but if you are familiar with the nutrition data of other sub shops, you can make educated guesses about any restaurant's food.

Healthy Choices

First, exercise portion control and choose a 6-inch, small, or regular-size sandwich. If a smaller sandwich isn't an option, save the other half for another meal or split it with a dining companion. The healthier meats are turkey, smoked turkey, roast beef, and ham. Keep the cheese to a minimum. Instead, load on the veggies, like lettuce, tomatoes, cucumbers, onions, and peppers. If you like some zip to your meal, toss on some hot peppers.

Complement your sandwich with some crunch from a bag of pretzels or popcorn. Better yet, order a side or garden salad. Salads are an alternative to sub sandwiches. Most menus offer the standards: garden, chef, grilled chicken, turkey, club, Greek, and tossed salads with a scoop of premixed, mayo-laden tuna fish, chicken, or seafood. The healthiest salads are garden, grilled chicken, turkey, and Greek. Don't forget to order the dressing on the side and request some vinegar to thin it out. Get more help with your salad choices in Chapter 13: Salad Style—Bar, Entrée, or Side.

Tolerable Choices

If you've got a few more calories and a bit more fat to spare, you can choose a steak sandwich with onions, peppers, or mushrooms, but avoid the steak and cheese. A sautéed veggie with cheese sandwich is tolerable, as is a meatball sub with no cheese.

Worst Choices

As was true in the delicatessens, there are some choices to avoid: bologna, all types of salami, mortadella, pepperoni, cheese, sausage and peppers, and steak and cheese. A few other sandwich fillers to avoid are eggplant, chicken, and veal parmigiana. They may sound healthy, but they are breaded, deep-fried, and smothered in cheese.

Food-Court Eateries

Today's food courts aren't just in shopping malls. You can now find food courts in airports, universities, hospitals, and other institutions as well. They usually offer several fast-food restaurants (see Chapter 11: Fast-Food Style); dessert places, like Cinnabon and TCBY; smoothie shops; and some ethnic choices, like Chinese, Middle Eastern, Mexican, pizza, and maybe even sushi. Airport food courts often offer a few health-focused kiosks with premade salads, sandwiches, and fresh fruit—but expect to pay a premium for it.

Food courts offer several advantages. Food is served quickly— you simply stand in line, order, and eat. If you dine with a group, everyone has an opportunity to pick his or her favorite cuisine and still eat together. Unfortunately, you can also become overwhelmed by the visual and taste stimuli, and even a carefully planned meal can go by the wayside when you are confronted with so many choices. Remain confident in your choice. Know where you will eat and what you will order. Do not let your eyes wander.

Healthy, Tolerable, and Worst Choices

Look for places that serve fresh, unadulterated foods, like fruit cups, frozen yogurt, salads, sub sandwiches, stuffed pita pockets, Greek salads, or stuffed baked potatoes with chili or sautéed vegetables. Steer clear of the fried foods: fried chicken or fish, French fries, deep-fried vegetables, double- and triple-decker burgers, and high-fat sandwich stuffings. Read the ethnic food chapters in Part III to pick up pointers for your favorite ethnic cuisines at the mall or the location of other food courts.

Typical Menu: Lighter Bites

✣ *Indicates preferred choices*

Soups

   New England clam chowder
  ✣ **Chili**
  ✣ **Vegetable soup**

✿ **Black bean**
　Cheesy broccoli
✿ **Chicken and wild rice**

Salads

Served with choice of dressing: blue cheese, thousand island, Italian, French, ranch, lemon-garlic, or low-calorie Italian. Always request the dressing on the side and use it sparingly. If your salad includes cheese, ask that it be left off or eat little of it.

✿ **House salad** (lettuce topped with peppers, mushrooms, cucumbers, and tomatoes)
✿ **Greek salad** (a bed of lettuce topped with crumbled feta cheese, red onions, and Greek olives)
✿ **Chef salad** (a bed of greens topped with ham, turkey, Swiss cheese, tomatoes, and cucumbers)
　Tuna, chicken, or seafood salad (a bed of greens with tomato, green peppers, and bean sprouts topped with a scoop of tuna, chicken, or seafood salad)
✿ **Roasted chicken salad** (sliced roasted chicken served on a bed of romaine lettuce, sliced tomato, and cucumber)

Cold Sandwiches

✿ **Smoked turkey**
✿ **Roast beef**
　Egg salad
　Chicken salad
　Tuna salad
　Seafood salad
　Hot pastrami
✿ **Corned beef (lean)**
✿ **Ham**

Ham and cheese
Club sandwich (choice of turkey or roast beef)

Hot Sandwiches

Reuben (corned beef served with cheese and sauerkraut and topped with thousand island dressing)

✿ **Hamburger**

Grilled cheese

✿ **Grilled chicken breast**

Bacon, lettuce, and tomato

Grilled hot dog

Tuna melt (a scoop of tuna salad with melted mozzarella cheese)

✿ **Meatball** (hold the cheese)

✿ **Vegetarian** (roasted vegetables covered with fresh mozzarella cheese)

Bread Choices

✿ **Submarine roll** (choose a 6-inch or half sandwich, and request whole grain if possible)

White

✿ **Whole-grain**

✿ **Pumpernickel**

Focaccia

Kaiser roll

Croissant

✿ **Whole grain wrap**

✿ **Spinach wrap**

Combinations

✿ **Soup and salad** (a cup of soup served with a house or spinach salad)

✿ **Soup or salad with a half-sandwich** (a cup of any soup or salad served with half a cold sandwich)

Side Orders

French fries
✿ Tabbouleh
Potato salad
✿ Garden salad
Potato chips
Corn chips
Onion rings
✿ Coleslaw (OK if it is vinegar-based; skip it if it is creamy)
✿ Popcorn
✿ Pretzels

Desserts

Chocolate-chip cookies
Chocolate cake
Apple pie
✿ Fresh fruit cup (usually large enough to split)
✿ Fresh fruit (banana, orange, apple)
✿ Frozen lowfat yogurt

Low-Calorie Sample Meal

Roasted chicken salad
(dressing on the side)
Quantity: 3 oz. meat (lean)
Dressing (on the side)
Quantity: 2 tablespoons
Tabbouleh with lemon-herb
dressing
Quantity: ½ cup
Apple (brought from home)
Quantity: 1 small
Mineral water
Quantity: 10 oz

> **NUTRITION SUMMARY**
> 425 calories
> Carb: 50 g, 46%
> Fat: 10 g, 21%
> Protein: 35 g, 33%
> Cholesterol: 73 mg
> Sodium: 862 mg

Moderate-Calorie Sample Meal

Bean and barley soup
Quantity: 1 cup
Ham and cheese sandwich
Quantity: ½
Potato chips
Quantity: ½ bag (share or split
between two meals)

> **NUTRITION SUMMARY**
> 555 calories
> Carb: 72 g, 52%
> Fat: 20 g, 32%
> Protein: 22 g, 16%
> Cholesterol: 34 mg
> Sodium: 1860 mg (750
> accounted for by soup)

13

Salad Style—Bar, Entrée or Side

How many times have you spoken these virtuous words: "You guys have your burgers and fries. I'll just make a trip to the salad bar," or "I'm watching my waistline. I'll just have the Cobb salad." Unfortunately, making a well-intended trip (or trips, more likely) an all-you-can-eat salad bar or ordering a healthy-sounding salad can result in shockingly high-fat, high-calorie meals if you aren't careful.

Salad bars had their heyday back in the late 1990s and early 2000s. Almost every category of restaurants, from steak houses to fast-food establishments, offered them. However, many began to question the hygiene of self-service salad bars, and their up-keep is labor intensive. As a result, there are far fewer salad bars today, but you will still encounter them at some steak houses, seafood and family restaurants.

Salad bars are also still common in supermarkets, where many in the lunch and dinner crowd are looking for a quick and inexpensive meal. You'll also find salad bars in hospital, employee, and university cafeterias. They are a diverse lot: some offer simple salad fixings and a few extras, and others are stocked for a feeding frenzy, with raw vegetables, cheese, legumes, canned fruit, pasta salad, tuna and chicken salad, fruit ambrosia, baked goods, puddings, and more. Obviously, if there's more to choose from, there's more danger of making poor choices.

As salad bars have waned, packaged and plated entrée salads have become more popular. You can order an entrée salad, such as a Cobb, chef or Caesar, at many types of restaurants. In the fast-food sector Wendy's led the pack, introducing its line of entrée salads in the early 2000s. Others followed suit, and today, most fast food chains offer garden salads, side salads, and three to five types of entrée salads. Entrée salads are also common at family-fare and soup 'n' sandwich restaurants, such as Ruby Tuesday, Panera Bread, Au Bon Pain, and Applebee's.

The word "salad" brings to mind visions of lettuce, spinach, tomatoes, and peppers. However, in and among those healthy salad bar choices lurks pasta salad, potato salad, vegetables marinated in oil, pepperoni, cheeses, and other high-fat foods that boost calories.

Perhaps most damaging is the salad dressing. The primary American favorites—blue cheese and thousand island—contain more than 70 calories per tablespoon. When the salad bar is your entrée, you're likely to pour on at least a few tablespoons of dressing. Under the guise of a "healthy" food choice, a meal from the salad bar can actually be higher in fat and calories than a burger and fries.

However, if you can approach the salad bar or order an entrée salad with a plan and control the choice and amount of the salad dressing, salads can be a winner. A trip to a salad bar or an entrée salad can be a nutritionally complete lunch or dinner. A side garden salad can add in some vegetables and help you limit higher-fat items that usually accompany sandwiches or burgers, like potato chips or French fries.

Nutrition Snapshot

The following nutrition snapshot is intended to provide you with the nutrition numbers for a handful of commonly served entrée and side salads served at a wide variety of restaurants. Some salads are dressed, and others are not—you'll see that salad dressings can be a minefield of added fat and calories. Other high-fat items, such as cheese, bacon bits, nuts, and fried chicken, also rack up the fat and calories. On page 134, check out The Lowdown on Salad Dressings chart. In it and the nutrition snapshot chart, you'll see nutrition numbers that range from mind-blowing to healthy. Use them to learn about the nutrition profile of your current favorite salads. If necessary, change your favorites to healthier alternatives.

Menu Item	Calories	Carbohy-drate (g)	Fat (g)	Saturated Fat (g)	*Trans* Fat (g)	Sodium (mg)
Caesar Salad with Dressing (Panera Bread) 10 oz	440	25	32	9	0	850
Choose a different salad with more vegetables and less cheese and dressing. Order dressing on the side and use it sparingly.						
Grilled Chicken Caesar Salad with Dressing (Panera Bread) 14 oz	560	26	34	9	0	1207
Move on to another salad with more vegetables and less fat. Order dressing on the side and use it sparingly.						
Grilled Salmon Salad without Dressing (Panera Bread) 13.5 oz	340	32	14	3	0	820
A healthy choice.						
Asian Salad with Crispy Chicken without Dressing (McDonald's) 13 oz	380	33	17	3	2	1030
Request grilled, instead of fried, chicken on your salad.						
Side Salad without Dressing (McDonald's) 3 oz	20	4	0	0	0	10
A healthy choice.						
Chef's Salad without Dressing (Denny's) 18 oz	360	17	17	7	0	1680
Ask for some substitutions—more turkey and less ham and cheese—to lower the saturated fat and sodium counts.						

Menu Item	Calories	Carbohy-drate (g)	Fat (g)	Saturated Fat (g)	*Trans* Fat (g)	Sodium (mg)
Martha's Vineyard without Dressing (Arby's) 12 oz	276	24	8	4	0	451
A healthy choice.						
Grilled Chicken without Dressing (Dairy Queen)	240	12	10	5	0	950
A healthy choice.						
Strawberry Poppyseed with Dressing (Panera Bread)	200	33	3	0	0	240
A healthy choice.						
Oven-Roasted Chicken without Dressing (Subway)	140	11	3	.5	0	400
A healthy choice.						
Tomato and Fresh Mozzarella with Dressing (Panera Bread)	720	58	43	20	1.5	950
Enjoy the tomatoes, skip the mozzarella, and request the dressing on the side.						

The Lowdown on Salad Dressings

Salad Dressing (amount—2 tbsp/1 oz)	Calories	Carbohy-drate (g)	Fat (g)	Saturated Fat (g)	*Trans* Fat (g)	Choles-terol (mg)	Sodium (mg)
Regular							
Newman's Own Creamy Caesar (McDonald's)	80	2	9	2	0	10	250
Creamy Caesar (Burger King)	105	2	11	2	0	14	305
Newman's Own Southwest (McDonald's)	75	4	6	0	0	15	250
Honey Mustard (Burger King)	135	11	12	2	0	10	270
Creamy Ranch (Burger King)	95	2	10	2	0	10	280
Italian (Pizza Hut)	70	1	8	1.5	0	0	180

Salad Dressing (amount—2 tbsp/1 oz)	Calories	Carbohy-drate (g)	Fat (g)	Saturated Fat (g)	*Trans* Fat (g)	Choles-terol (mg)	Sodium (mg)
Raspberry Vinaigrette (Arby's)	97	9	7	1	0	0	194
Balsamic Vinaigrette (Panera Bread)	95	7	8	1	0	0	185
Thousand Island (Pizza Hut)	60	5	6	1	0	5	110
French Dressing (Pizza Hut)	75	5	7	1	0	0	90
Blue Cheese (Domino's)	115	1	12	2.5	0	15	225
Light/Low/Reduced Calorie							
Lowfat Italian (McDonald's)	40	6	2	0	0	0	510
Lite Italian (Pizza Hut)	70	5	5	1	0	0	510
Reduced-Sugar Asian Sesame Vinaigrette (Panera Bread)	60	3	5	.5	0	0	260
Lite Ranch (Pizza Hut)	60	2	6	1	0	16	260
Nonfat							
Ranch (Burger King)	30	8	0	0	0	0	370
Italian (KFC)	20	3	0	0	0	0	200
Italian (Denny's)	15	3	0	0	0	0	390
Poppyseed (Panera Bread)	15	4	0	0	0	0	100
Raspberry (Panera Bread)	25	6	0	0	0	0	47
Alternatives/Dressing Diluters							
Vinegar (any type)	3	1	0	0	0	0	0
Lemon or Lime Juice	11	3	0	0	0	0	0

Salad Bar "Won't Power"

Because the slew of items available on a large salad bar can be overwhelming, you need a dose of "won't power." If you are extremely hungry, hitting the salad bar can be disastrous. If your won't power can't resist a tempting salad bar, stay at the table and order from the menu. In some lower-priced steak houses—

where salad bars should be called food bars—you'd be much better off ordering a small steak, baked potato, and vegetables and skipping the salad bar altogether.

Here are a few strategies to cure wavering self-discipline. Survey the salad bar carefully without a plate, and if you're with a sympathetic friend, you can coerce him or her to make the trip, and ask your dining companion to exercise portion control for you. If you're alone, use a smaller plate. If you use a smaller plate, you have less space to load the food—portion control at its simplest level. Limit yourself to only one trip.

Manage the Salad Bar

Rather than choosing with your eyes and taste buds, make decisions with your nutrition and health goals in mind. Think about what foods you really need, and how much you really need.

Nutritionally speaking, salad bars can be great as part of a meal or as an entire meal. You can find plenty of healthy carbohydrates with lots of fiber and little fat. Filling up on greens and vegetables helps you keep the protein down. If you know which items are high in fat and cholesterol, you can keep them to a minimum.

When you're watching your sodium intake, salad bars can range from great to disastrous—again it's a matter of what foods you choose to eat. Vegetables are extremely low in sodium, but salad "mix-ins," such as macaroni salad, coleslaw, ham, olives, pickles, and croutons, can max out the sodium.

The Salad-Bar Calorie Counter on pages 137–140 divides common salad bar items into categories based on their calorie content. The best advice at the salad bar, no matter what your nutrition priorities are, is to load up on the veggies—greens, to-matoes, cucumbers, peppers, onions, mushrooms, raw broccoli, and carrots. Fill your plate with raw vegetables, which give you plenty of crunches and bites with few calories. Croutons, crackers, pita pockets, and hard-to-resist fresh baked breads are also common and are okay as long as you don't go overboard with the portions. Some lower-calorie protein options include plain tuna (not tuna salad), cubed ham (not ham salad), hard-boiled eggs (whole or chopped), feta cheese, and cottage cheese (just a little, since most salad bars only offer full-fat varieties). Remember, the ham and feta cheese are high in sodium. Tuna, chicken, potato, and seafood salad mixed with mayonnaise are loaded with fat and should be avoided. Chunks of cheese and pepperoni contain more calories from fat than protein.

Marinated beets, marinated mixed vegetables, mushrooms, three-bean salads, vinegar-based coleslaw, and mixed fruit salads are fine, but take small quantities (about ¼ to ½ cup), especially if you closely monitor calories, fat, and sodium.

Another group of foods that can add on calories are the so-called "salad bar accessories." These little temptations include nuts, raisins, seeds, Chinese noodles, olives, and bacon bits. A little of this and that can rack up calories fast. Use them sparingly.

Salad-Bar Calorie Counter

Low-Calorie Vegetables (mainly raw)

(approx. 25 calories per cup)

- broccoli
- cabbage (red or green)
- cauliflower
- celery
- cucumbers
- endive

- lettuce (all types)
- onions, raw (all types)
- peppers (all types)
- radishes
- sauerkraut (high in sodium)
- spinach (raw)
- sprouts (all types)
- summer squash, raw
- watercress
- zucchini, raw

Higher-Calorie Vegetables

(approx. 25 calories per ½ cup)

- artichokes, canned (not the variety that is marinated in oil, which is higher in calories)
- beets, canned (plain, not pickled)
- carrots, raw
- tomatoes, raw

Salad Bar "Accessories"

(see calories per tablespoon to the right of each item)

- pickles, 2–5
- hot peppers, 2–5
- raisins, 10
- Chinese noodles, 20
- bacon bits, 27
- sunflower seeds, 47
- olives, green or black, 50
- peanuts, 50
- sesame seeds, 52

Starches

(60–100 calories per ½ cup)

- chickpeas (garbanzo beans)
- kidney beans
- green peas
- croutons (commercial)
- crackers (4–6)
- bread (1 slice, or 1 oz.)
- pita pocket (½ of a 6 to 8-inch loaf)

Lean Protein (meat)

(40–80 calories per ounce)

- plain tuna
- cottage cheese
- egg (hard boiled)
- ham
- feta cheese

Higher-Fat Protein

(100 calories per ounce)

- cheese
- pepperoni

Salad Bar Mixtures

(35–50 calories per ¼ cup)

- marinated/pickled beets
- marinated artichoke hearts
- three-bean salad
- assorted marinated vegetables

- marinated mushrooms
- pasta salad, oil-based
- gelatin with fruit
- fruit salad

Salad Bar Mixtures

(50–80 calories per ¼ cup)

- tuna salad
- chicken salad
- seafood salad
- corn relish
- macaroni salad
- potato salad
- fruit ambrosia
- pasta salad, mayonnaise-based

Entrée Salads

When you are looking for a salad entrée, make sure your choice is well padded with lots of veggies. Make sure the menu description includes lots of greens, cucumbers, tomatoes, carrots, and similar low-calorie vegetables. Always be mindful of the higher-calorie, higher-fat ingredients that are often included.

Consider a Cobb salad, which contains avocado, blue cheese, and bacon—three fat-packed ingredients. The fat in the avocado is healthier, but the bacon and blue cheese are high in saturated fat. Next, think about the Caesar salad. The romaine lettuce and even the meats that are added, like shrimp or chicken, aren't the issue. The Parmesan cheese and creamy Caesar dressing send the calories skyrocketing. The good news is that you can control the amounts of these ingredients on your salads by telling the server to leave them out or serve them on the side.

Look for salads that mainly contain healthy salad items— grilled chicken or shrimp, ham, smoked turkey, beans, peas, etc. Next, be creative. If you think a particular salad is basically a healthy choice but contains one or two ingredients that aren't, ask that they be left off, sprinkled sparingly, or served on the side. You can also consider sharing an entrée-size salad. As portions for all restaurant foods have grown, even salads are often large enough for two people. You may also ask for a take-home container when you order your meal. Immediately after it is served, place half the salad in the container, where it won't tempt you—but it'll be a great lunch or dinner the next day!

Last, but not least, choose a salad dressing that doesn't top the fat and calorie scale, and ask that it be served on the side. Ask for some vinegar or lemon juice to dilute the dressing as well. See more suggestions in the next section, The Lowdown on Salad Dressings, to whittle down the calories in salad dressing.

The Lowdown on Salad Dressings

By far the biggest culprit in adding abundant and hidden calories is salad dressing. The Lowdown on Salad Dressings chart on page 134 details the numbers in black and white, and the section Dress with Less Dressing on page 143 also provides some helpful tips.

Most restaurants, cafeterias, and supermarket salad bars primarily stock regular commercial salad dressing. These include oil-based choices, like Italian and balsamic vinaigrette, as well as creamier options, like French, honey mustard, thousand island, and blue cheese. Very few chain restaurants make their salad dressings from scratch; usually only independently owned family or fine-dining restaurants bother to do so. However, most restaurants do stock olive oil and a variety of vinegars, because they are common kitchen ingredients. Request these two ingredients and fresh ground pepper, too, and you've got the healthiest and freshest salad dressing possible.

Most oil-based commercial salad dressings contain soybean or cottonseed oil or a combination of the two. Some salad dressings also contain canola or olive oil to boost their levels of monounsaturated fats. Regular salad dressings have about 60–80 calories per level tablespoon—and most people aren't leveling those tablespoons. In addition to the calories, creamy dressings may contain mayonnaise, sour cream, and/or cheese, which can add saturated or *trans* fat and/or cholesterol.

These days, it's common to find at least one or more low-fat, reduced-calorie, or nonfat salad dressing available in restaurants, especially in fast-food outlets. They range from 15–30 calories per tablespoon. That's half or less than half the calories of regular dressing. You should be aware that some lower-calorie and lowfat salad dressings deliver even more sodium and carbohydrates than regular salad dressings. If you take the fat out, you've got to replace it with something. That "something" usually ends up being carbohydrate-based fat replacers, sugars, and high-sodium ingredients. Four tablespoons (¼ cup, which is the usual serving size in a package of fast-food salad dressing) of either a regular or reduced-calorie dressing can contain as much as 500 milligrams of sodium, and some nonfat salad dressings have even more.

This does not mean you have to eat your salad without dressing. There are many healthy options. However, if you are used to seeing a pool of dressing in your dish after finishing a salad, learning to use less dressing is a great move in the right direction.

Dress with Less Dressing

Using one or more of these tips can help you cut your calories, total fat, saturated fat (depending on the dressing), and sodium. You'll quickly realize that using less dressing helps you enjoy the various tastes of your salad more.

- Always order dressing on the side. This puts you in control instead of the kitchen.
- Drizzle instead of pouring. If you want to use your favorite dressing, fine—just use less of it. When you get a large packet of salad dressing from a fast-food restaurant, drizzle slowly and gingerly. Mix up your salad in between drizzles to see if your salad is sufficiently coated.
- Instead of putting dressing directly on your salad, dip your fork in it before assembling each bite of salad. You'll get the taste of the dressing and use far less of it.
- Use half your usual serving of your favorite dressing and thin it with vinegar, lemon juice, or water.
- Think about simply mixing your own salad dressing with olive oil and vinegar—the healthiest salad dressing combo because it contains healthy oils and no sodium.

14

Fine-Dining Style

Today, upscale restaurants offer a wider variety of foods than ever before. Fine dining has evolved from standard American fare served graciously on a linen-covered table to diverse fusions of cuisines. A fine-dining establishment might boast a blend of French and Vietnamese food or a mix of various Asian or Middle Eastern cuisines. These menus expose you to foods, cooking styles, and culinary techniques from around the world.

One great fine-dining concept for those seeking portion control are tapas or small plates. The concept involves ordering a variety of small appetizer-sized portions of various dishes and sharing them with dining companions. "Tapas" is a Spanish word meaning "lids." The name originated from pieces of bread or ham that were used to cover wineglasses and keep the flies out. As it turns out, these tapas made tasty appetizers as well. Today, you'll find tapas-style menus for many cuisines, including a fusion of tastes from around the world.

In the world of fine dining, there is also a move toward serving organic and/or locally grown produce and promoting sustainable agriculture. Alice Waters, owner of the highly regarded Chez Panisse restaurant in Berkeley, California, has pioneered the movement.

Big cities around the country have upscale restaurants with nearly any cuisine you can think of, from Asian to Middle Eastern and more. For detailed information on upscale dining for each ethnic cuisine, read the chapter dedicated to that particular style of cuisine. Since estimating portions in these restaurants is more challenging, review the strategies for portion control in Chapter 5. Remember to check the menu of upscale restaurants carefully before you ask for a table: There are still plenty that prepare most of their foods using traditional French cooking methods, which can mean drenching foods in rich béchamel, béarnaise, or beurre blanc sauces.

Several of the changes that have happened in fine dining serve the health conscious well. A wide variety of foods and tastes means a wider array of nutrients. Smaller servings make it easier to eat less without compromising on variety and taste. Last, fine-dining restaurants are more willing than ever before to handle your special requests.

No matter what cuisine you choose, you have different expectations about a dining experience in an upscale restaurant. You expect a tablecloth, a full water glass, and an attentive wait staff. Unlike less formal spots, you'll linger over your meal for as long as three hours to enjoy each morsel and relish the relaxing environment.

The Menu Profile

The first question your server will probably ask is, "What can I bring you to drink?" Many fine-dining meals are accompanied by a cocktail before dinner, wine with dinner, and a cordial at the end of the evening. Such a liberal flow of alcohol can quickly add up to hundreds of calories. Figure out a plan for your alcohol consumption that works best for you. Is a preliminary glass of wine sufficient, or are you best off with a club soda with lime before your meal and a glass of wine with your meal? Gather more tips and tactics to manage your alcohol consumption in Chapter 8.

Once your beverage order is in, you may receive a small taste-bud teaser and/or a bread assortment and accompanying spreads. It's often hard to resist, but set limits. If the bread is excellent, allow yourself one piece, preferably without butter. If you must moisten your bread, ask the server to bring you what Rachael Ray calls EVOO—extra virgin olive oil. If you can take it or leave it, bank your calories for a wonderful starch or dessert. Next, contemplate your dinner order.

Appetizers and soups are often laden with fat, but there are usually a few healthy choices. When it comes to appetizers, look for unadulterated and unfried seafood or vegetables, such as a marinated ceviche, a shrimp cocktail, or blanched asparagus. Appetizers are perfect for sharing because they are served in small quantities.

Look for healthy choices on the soup list, such as broth, to-mato, bean, or vegetable-based types. They're usually served by the bowl, which presents another opportunity to split a serving down the middle. Ask your server to divide the serving in the kitchen. Stay away from the creamy soups and bisques because of their high fat content. If any item is not well explained on the menu, ask questions.

Be creative with the menu and select an appetizer, a salad, and a soup to create a portion-controlled meal. Another strategy for portion control is splitting each course—from appetizer to dessert—with a dining companion. This strategy makes room for lots of tastes but not lots of food.

An excellent strategy for a party of three or more is to eat "family-style." Consider ordering fewer entrées than there are people in your party. Usually two entrées can serve three people.

Put the entrées in the center of the table and ask for side plates—you can create your own tapas.

Next up are salads. A healthy salad is a great alternative to an appetizer or soup. Look for salads full of healthy greens, low-calorie vegetables, and interesting and unique ingredients like endive, jicama, radicchio, beets, pears, apples, and nuts. Be cautious with salad dressing. Select a vinaigrette or other oil-based dressing on the side, or ask the server to bring you olive oil and vinegar. Ask that high-fat salad toppings, such as bacon, croutons, and cheeses, be left off or used sparingly.

The entrée usually gets the most attention. Will it be chicken, duck, lamb, or shrimp? No matter which entrée you choose, you'll probably be served a portion that is at least six to eight ounces—about twice what you should eat. Be ready to practice portion control and menu creativity. Split or share dishes to minimize the amount of protein, request a to-go container, or leave some on your plate. Think about choosing lower-fat protein sources like fish, shellfish, and chicken—as long as they don't hit the deep fryer or get soaked in butter before arriving your plate.

Consider the following description of Chicken Kiev: a breast of chicken filled with herb butter and garlic cheese, served with butter sauce. Compare this with the Chicken and Vegetable Sauté: diced chicken breast sautéed in olive oil and served with sun-dried tomatoes, herbs, and asparagus. Neither dish is non-fat, but the latter is certainly a lower-fat and healthier choice. Seafood medleys, such as cioppino and bouillabaisse, offer healthfully prepared fish. Grilled, poached, or similar preparations of fish that keep the fat low are healthy choices.

Seafood and chicken are often healthier choices, but unadulterated beef, lamb, or veal can be good bets too. If you order meat, stick with a small cut—"petite," "queen," "filet mignon," and "8-ounce" are common descriptions of smaller servings.

Even these smaller cuts can be plenty for two people. Search for dishes that mix meats with starches or vegetables, as they will usually contain less protein.

Always select a leaner cut of meat. Filet mignon (also called tenderloin) and sirloin are leaner cuts than ribeye, porterhouse, T-bone, or prime rib. Veal is commonly breaded and sautéed prior to cooking, but a broiled veal chop is worth considering. Some cuts of lamb can be high in fat, but the preparation is usually broiling or grilling, which doesn't add much fat. If there's visible fat on the meat when it arrives, take some time to trim it off. Loin lamb chops are the best choice.

Duck is traditionally served with the skin intact, which means that it is high in fat. However, many upscale restaurants now offer sliced duck breast, which is quite lean and skinless. Light fruit sauces or glazes are often served with duck breast; order them on the side and use them in small amounts if they are high in sugar or fat.

An increasing number of upscale restaurants now offer vegetarian entrées. Consider them a good way to cut back on your protein intake; they may include pasta dishes, Chinese stir-fries, or grilled vegetable platters. Be wary of vegetarian entrées that are loaded with fat and cheese.

You can also avoid meat by ordering à la carte appetizers, soups, salads, and side items, and skipping the entrée, or reduce your protein by splitting one vegetarian entrée and one protein-dense entrée between two or even three people.

A starch is usually included with the entrée or available à la carte. Look for low- or nonfat starches: baked potatoes, red potatoes, rice, couscous, millet, barley, or quinoa. If you are ordering potatoes, ask that the cheese, butter, and sour cream to be served on the side.

If your meal includes vegetables (and hopefully it will), ask how they are prepared. Make sure that cream, cheese, sour cream, and rich sauces like hollandaise are not involved in the preparation. Steamed vegetables are healthiest. Sautéed, grilled, and roasted veggies probably have some oil added. If no vegetables come with your entrée, order them à la carte and specify how you want them prepared. You may even request a double order so you get more than a few pieces.

Most upscale dining establishments have impressive and tempting dessert menus. Needless to say, they are often decadent as well. However, these are often great opportunities to spend the dessert calories you've been saving up. Go ahead, but realize that maybe a taste or two of a sweet is all you really need to satisfy your sweet tooth. Share a dessert with several dining companions. Many fine-dining restaurants offer fresh fruit desserts, such as berries with crème fraîche and liqueur. Hold the crème fraîche but let them drizzle the liqueur—it's fat-free.

The length of time you linger, the dangerous foods placed on the table with even ordering them (bread and butter), the quantity of food that is served, the more elaborate preparations, the higher-fat foods, the alcohol, and the tempting desserts—all these factors can add up to make upscale continental dining more difficult. However, the same tips and tactics of healthy restaurant eating in other establishments apply here. Use them to your advantage: Have a game plan in mind; exercise portion control from the moment you begin to order; make special requests; and know when to say "enough."

Pick and choose which food courses you want and forget about the others. Avoid prix-fixe or table d'hôte menus that might make you feel compelled to eat something because it's included. Focus on the pleasure of the special occasion and/or the restaurant's pleasant environment. Luxuriating in its ambiance helps take the importance off the food and places it instead on the company and the surroundings.

▷ Green Flag Words

Ingredients

△ balsamic, raspberry, or any vinegar

△ light vinaigrette

△ roasted peppers

△ sun-dried tomatoes

△ herbs and spices

△ onion, garlic, shallots

△ grains—barley, couscous, millet, polenta, quinoa, cracked wheat, wheat berries

△ rice—brown, wild

△ salsa—fruit or vegetable-based

△ chipotle peppers or sauces

△ olives, olive oil

△ mustards

Cooking Methods/Menu Descriptions/Names

△ blackened

△ Cajun

△ wine sauce—red or white (make sure not a cream sauce)

△ mustard sauce—(make sure not a cream sauce)

△ tomato, garlic, and herb sauce

△ fruit sauce

△ roasted

△ steamed

△ poached

△ grilled, grilled on mesquite or hickory chips

△ marinated

△ en brochette (on skewer)

△ en papillote (in parchment package)

△ petite or queen size

△ au jus (with juice of meat)

▶ Red Flag Words

Ingredients

▼ melted cheese

▼ cheese—blue, goat, mozzarella, feta, Parmesan

▼ butter, drawn butter, cream

▼ bacon

▼ pancetta

▼ sausage

▼ pistachio, orange, herb, garlic butter

▼ hollandaise, rémoulade, mornay sauce (or any other white sauces and mayonnaise-based sauces)

▼ sour cream

▼ crème fraîche

▼ whipped cream

▼ nuts (large amounts are not OK, but small amounts are)

Cooking Methods/Menu Descriptions/Names

▼ creamy mushroom sauce

▼ cheese sauce

▼ au gratin

▼ stuffed with seasoned bread crumbs

▼ Wellington

▼ Stroganoff

▼ garlic and herbed cream sauce

▼ casserole (usually has butter, cream and/or cheese and bread crumb topping)

▼ wrapped in bacon, phyllo dough, puffed pastry

▼ served in pastry shell

At the Table

- ▼ butter
- ▼ olive oil
- ▼ sour cream
- ▼ salad dressing
- ▼ high-fat sauces

Special Requests

- ◆ "Would you serve the salad dressing on the side?"
- ◆ "Can you leave the cheese off the salad?"
- ◆ "Could you serve the sauce on the side?"
- ◆ "Could I get some olive oil and vinegar, balsamic vinegar or lemon wedges for my salad rather than the dressing?"
- ◆ "May I have some Dijon mustard or salsa for my potato?"
- ◆ "Please don't add butter or sour cream to my potato. Instead, bring it on the side."
- ◆ "Please don't add butter to my steak before it's served."
- ◆ "Could I ask you how this is prepared?"
- ◆ "What is _____ (unfamiliar ingredient)?"
- ◆ "Is it possible to have these vegetables steamed instead of sautéed?"
- ◆ "Please bring my appetizer/soup when you bring the others their main courses."
- ◆ "Could we get an extra plate to split this appetizer (or entrée)?"
- ◆ "We will share this entrée. Can you split it in the kitchen?"
- ◆ "Can you bring several extra forks? We are going to share this dessert."
- ◆ "May I have this wrapped up to take home?"

Typical Menu: Upscale Continental Style

✵ *Indicates preferred choices*

Appetizers

Mussels au gratin (mussels in garlic butter sauce with cheese topping)

✵ **Marinated grilled shrimp** (marinated and grilled quarter pound of shrimp, served with cocktail dipping sauce)

Fried calamari (rounds of squid breaded with herbs and fried to perfection)

Stuffed mushrooms (prepared with herbs and seasoned bread crumbs, topped with rosemary in cream sauce)

Pâté de la maison (pâté de foie gras, served with toast points)

Escargots (snails served with garlic, herbs, butter sauce)

✵ **Vegetable mélange** with mustard sauce (freshly cut raw vegetables served in a lettuce cup with curry mustard sauce)

✵ **Grilled asparagus** (with lemon sauce)

✵ **Artichoke hearts** with feta cheese (artichoke hearts marinated and sautéed in olive oil, topped with crumbled feta cheese)

✵ **Tuna or steak tartare** (raw thinly sliced tuna served with soy sauce, wasabi, and pickled ginger)

Soups

Ask that any cheeses or breads be deleted from your serving.

✵ **French onion** (traditional style, served in a crock with melted Gruyère cheese)

Lobster bisque (the meat of a fresh lobster blended with cream and spices)

✿ **Butternut squash** (puréed butternut squash with bits of steamed lobster)

✿ **Gazpacho** (cold tomato-based soup of assorted puréed fresh vegetables)

Cream of broccoli (creamy-based soup with puréed fresh broccoli heads)

Salads

✿ **House salad** (mixture of romaine and Bibb lettuce, with red onions, red bell peppers, and sprouts, with raspberry vinaigrette dressing)

✿ **Endive stuffed with diced beets and goat cheese** (leaves of fresh endive stuffed with roasted beets and topped with crumbled goat cheese)

✿ **Baby field greens** (mixture of baby field greens and radicchio, endive, and jicama, topped with creamy anchovy dressing)

Spinach salad (fresh spinach, topped with sliced mushrooms, egg, and bacon bits with hot bacon dressing)

✿ **Marinated tomatoes** (sliced tomatoes marinated with red onions in olive oil and balsamic vinegar, topped with crumbled feta cheese)

Entrées

Most of these dishes are enough for two to split or to ask for a take home container early in the meal.

Meat

Beef Wellington (filet of beef covered with thin layer of goose liver pâté and wrapped in flaky pastry shell, topped with bordelaise sauce)

✱ **Petite filet mignon** (with sautéed cremini mushrooms and onions)

New York sirloin (12 ozs. grilled to your liking)

✱ **Marinated pork chop** (10 ozs. broiled in sherry and lemon herb sauce)

✱ **Rack of lamb** (roasted with a glaze of honey mustard sauce)

Veal Oscar (veal cutlet sautéed with lobster meat and asparagus, topped with hollandaise sauce)

Poultry

Chicken Kiev (boneless breast of chicken, filled with herb butter and cheese garlic, topped with butter sauce)

✱ **Chicken sauté** (sliced chicken breast sautéed with sun-dried tomatoes, asparagus, and herbs in olive oil)

Duck à l'orange (one-half a Long Island duckling grilled and basted with orange glaze)

✱ **Duck with raspberry sauce** (sliced breast of duck served with a light raspberry-lemon sauce)

Seafood

Stuffed shrimp (four jumbo shrimp stuffed with a blend of crabmeat and seasoned bread crumbs and baked and basted with garlic butter sauce)

✱ **Poached salmon** (with smoked tomato sauce and cilantro)

Dover sole (in champagne cream sauce)

✱ **Grilled tuna** (steak served with peach and mango salsa)

Seafood fettuccine (shrimp and scallops topped with basil cream sauce over fettuccine)

Other

✱ **Grilled vegetables and polenta cakes** (eggplant, zucchini, and red peppers grilled with basil and oregano and served with polenta cakes)

Cheese-stuffed tortellini (topped with sautéed broccoli and mushrooms)

✿ **Oriental stir-fry** (fresh garden vegetables, stir-fried in olive oil, tamari, garlic, and lemon and served over brown and wild rice)

Side Dishes

✿ **Rice pilaf**

✿ **Steamed red potatoes**

Fried potato puffs

✿ **Barley and sautéed mushrooms**

✿ **Baked potato**

Vegetables

✿ **Squash and zucchini** (sautéed in lemon herb butter)

✿ **Snow peas** (sautéed with red bell pepper strips)

Creamed spinach

✿ **Asparagus** (steamed and topped with hollandaise sauce—skip the hollandaise)

Desserts

✿ **Berries** (topped with crème fraîche and framboise)

Key lime pie

Peanut butter cheesecake

Chocolate raspberry cake (iced double fudge cake and filled with raspberry jam)

✿ **Fresh raspberries** (topped with Chambord liqueur)

Crème caramel (a light egg custard with caramel topping)

✿ **Sorbet trio** (small scoops of raspberry, lemon, and peach sorbet)

·················· ◆ **"May I Take Your Order?"** ▸ ··················

Low-Calorie Sample Meal

Shrimp, marinated and grilled (listed as appetizer but request as a main course)
Quantity: ¼ pound
Baby field greens (request the dressing on the side)
Quantity: 1–2 cups
Balsamic vinaigrette dressing (on the side)
Quantity: 1 tbsp.

> **NUTRITION SUMMARY**
> 580 calories
> Carb: 58 g, 40%
> Fat: 13 g, 20%
> Protein: 33 g, 23%
> Alcohol: 17%
> Cholesterol: 170 mg
> Sodium: 650 mg

Red potatoes, steamed (order as a side with no butter)
Quantity: 2
Berries (hold the crème fraîche)
Quantity: ½ cup
Wine
Quantity: 5 oz.

Moderate-Calorie Sample Meal

House salad (dressing on the side)
Quantity: 1–2 cups
Raspberry vinaigrette dressing (on the side)
Quantity: 2 tbsp.
Petite filet mignon
Quantity: 3 ozs. (½ order)
Oriental stir-fry with brown rice
Quantity: ½ order
Fresh raspberries with Chambord
Quantity: ½ cup

> **NUTRITION SUMMARY**
> 860 calories
> Carb: 95 g, 32%
> Fat: 31 g, 32%
> Protein: 34 g, 18%
> Alcohol: 6% calories
> Cholesterol: 67 mg
> Sodium: 790 mg

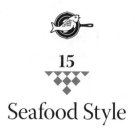

15

Seafood Style

Today, you'll find seafood on the menu in almost every restaurant. Fast-food spots offer fried fish sandwiches, sub shops and delis offer seafood and tuna salad, and family-fare restaurants offer many kinds of fried, poached, and grilled fish in everything from appetizers to main courses. There are countless independent seafood restaurants and several chains as well, including Bonefish Grill, Red Lobster, Joe's Crab Shack, and Legal Seafood.

Most seafood restaurants have an upscale ambience. An appetizer list might include marinated or fried calamari, grilled scallops, and perhaps a delightful ceviche (a particularly healthy choice). Main dishes will probably include shrimp, mahi mahi, Chilean sea bass or tuna prepared on the grill.

Most coastal areas have many independent and chain restaurants dedicated to seafood. Most offer a "raw bar" stocked with various types of oysters, steamed clams, and mussels. These restaurants usually serve a variety of fish prepared in multiple manners.

Seafood is also served in many ethnic restaurants. It is a staple of most Asian cuisines; Middle Eastern food features many delicious seafood preparations; and Mexican cuisine has marvelous seafood preparations. Check out the cuisine-specific chapters to learn more about each style.

Seafood preparations range from the very healthy, such as steamed, poached or grilled, to the unhealthy—deep-fried and drenched in fat. Consider the difference between an order of grilled swordfish and an order of fried clams with a mayonnaise-based tartar sauce. Even if the piece of swordfish is large enough for two, it's a much healthier choice, with omega-3 fat content.

Because of the increased demand for healthfully prepared finfish and shellfish, tasty cooking methods have evolved to please the nutrition-conscious. Seafood can be grilled on charcoal or flavored wood chips, seasoned with different combinations of spices, topped with a variety of wine- or mustard-based sauces, or paired with a variety of fruit or vegetable salsas. Sushi, which usually contains either raw or cooked seafood, has become more and more popular.

Seafood's Bottom Line: Eat More of It

Seafood has earned a gold star for health. The choices that receive the highest marks are high in omega-3 polyunsaturated fatty acids (EPA and DHA). Salmon is highest in omega-3s, but swordfish, mackerel, flounder, sole, trout, and herring are also good sources. Omega-3 fats reduce the risk of heart- and blood vessel-disease. When eaten in high enough levels, omega-3s can help decrease triglyceride levels, slightly lower blood pressure (if it is high), and decrease the growth rate of plaque on blood vessel walls. They have also been shown to reduce sudden death and death from coronary artery disease.

Health authorities recommend that Americans eat two or more servings of fish each week. The American Heart Association specifically recommends that adults eat 12 ounces of fish per week. When you eat fish you gain considerable health benefits. By choosing fish, you are also choosing to skip (displace, as the experts call it) more fattening foods, like red meats and cheeses. Therefore, people who choose fish more often eat less saturated and *trans* fat overall than people who do not.

Concerns About Contaminates

From time to time, you'll hear about unhealthy contaminants like mercury, polychlorinated biphenyls, and other chemicals, in seafood. The bottom line for most people is that the benefits of fish, as noted above, outweigh the risks. There are also ways to minimize your risks and still benefit from eating fish. According to the American Heart Association, shark, swordfish, king mackerel, and tilefish are among the varieties that can be high in mercury. Canned light tuna, salmon, pollack, and catfish are on the low end. Removing the skin and surface fat before cooking can mitigate the issue because the skin is where much of the contaminants are concentrated.

Women who are pregnant, planning to become pregnant, or breastfeeding and young children should avoid the types of fish that are considered high in mercury.

Nutrition Snapshot

The following nutrition snapshot is intended to provide you with the nutrition numbers for a handful of common seafood menu items. These items range from fish sandwiches served at fast-food burger chains to meals from fast-food fish restaurants and the sit-down establishments for which nutrition information is available. In the chart below, you'll see nutrition data that ranges from mind-blowing to healthy. Use them to learn about the nutrition profiles of your current favorite seafood meals. If necessary, change your favorites to healthier alternatives.

Menu Item	Calories	Carbohy-drate (g)	Fat (g)	Saturated Fat (g)	*Trans* Fat (g)	Sodium (mg)
Lobster Crab Cakes with Sauce—2 (Outback Steakhouse)	840	33	72	na	na	na

Don't get bitten by these crab cakes. Look at those fat grams! If you must, ask them to hold the sauce and request a red seafood cocktail sauce on the side.

Menu Item	Calories	Carbohy-drate (g)	Fat (g)	Saturated Fat (g)	*Trans* Fat (g)	Sodium (mg)
Clam Chowder (New England)—8 oz. (Denny's)	624	55	42	34	3.5	1474

Skip it. There are much healthier starters on the menu.

Menu Item	Calories	Carbohy-drate (g)	Fat (g)	Saturated Fat (g)	*Trans* Fat (g)	Sodium (mg)
Clam Chowder (New England)—8 oz. (Long John Silver's)	170	14	12	3	4	420

This chowder is lower in fat and calories than most.

Menu Item	Calories	Carbohy-drate (g)	Fat (g)	Saturated Fat (g)	*Trans* Fat (g)	Sodium (mg)
Blackened Codfish—8 oz. (Red Lobster)	270	na	7	1	na	560

Go for it. Reasonable 6 oz. portion cooked and blackened is a lowfat preparation.

Menu Item	Calories	Carbohy-drate (g)	Fat (g)	Saturated Fat (g)	*Trans* Fat (g)	Sodium (mg)
Broiled Salmon—8 oz (Red Lobster)	385	na	20	4	na	405

Go for it. Reasonable 6 oz. portion cooked. Request that no extra fat or oil should be added when cooking. This may cut the fat further.

Menu Item	Calories	Carbohy-drate (g)	Fat (g)	Saturated Fat (g)	*Trans* Fat (g)	Sodium (mg)
Fish Sandwich (Denny's)	589	30	30	5	4	1557

Opt for a lower-fat single hamburger instead.

Menu Item	Calories	Carbohy-drate (g)	Fat (g)	Saturated Fat (g)	*Trans* Fat (g)	Sodium (mg)
Baked Cod (Big Boy)	744	82	21	0	na	655

Skip it. Probably more breading than fish.

Menu Item	Calories	Carbohy-drate (g)	Fat (g)	Saturated Fat (g)	*Trans* Fat (g)	Sodium (mg)
Baked Shrimp Scampi Dinner (Captain D's)	590	43	34	na	11	790

Fat content is too high for this complete dinner.

Menu Item	Calories	Carbohy-drate (g)	Fat (g)	Saturated Fat (g)	*Trans* Fat (g)	Sodium (mg)
Shrimp Skewers Combo (Captain D's)	510	53	10	na	1	550

Great healthy choice.

Menu Item	Calories	Carbohy-drate (g)	Fat (g)	Saturated Fat (g)	*Trans* Fat (g)	Sodium (mg)
Fried Clams—8 oz	900	78	53	13	na	87

Skip. If you want clams, steamed is the way to go.

Menu Item	Calories	Carbohy-drate (g)	Fat (g)	Saturated Fat (g)	*Trans* Fat (g)	Sodium (mg)
Battered Fish—1 piece (Long John Silver's)	260	17	16	4	5	790

Skip. Go for broiled seafood.

Menu Item	Calories	Carbohy-drate (g)	Fat (g)	Saturated Fat (g)	*Trans* Fat (g)	Sodium (mg)
Mahi-Mahi—1 serving (Captain D's)	490	52	14	na	2	520
A healthy choice.						
Tilapia Combo—1 serving (Captain D's)	316	52	14	na	2	440
A healthy choice.						

The Menu Profile

Even with all this positive news about seafood, Americans aren't increasing their consumption of it. For years, levels of seafood consumption have been stable, and the types of fish that are eaten most frequently haven't changed either: shrimp, canned tuna, salmon, and pollack. Consider eating seafood more often and branching out to the varieties of seafood that offer you the most omega-3s.

All seafood ranges from about 30 to 60 calories per cooked ounce. The Seafood's Nutrition Assets and Liabilities chart on page 165 shows nutrition data for commonly served seafood. Cod, scallops, and monkfish are low in calories, and swordfish, salmon, and bluefish are higher in calories because they have a higher fat content. Most flatfish are lower in calories and fat than most cuts of red meats and some poultry.

A point of frequent misinformation is the belief that seafood is lower in dietary cholesterol than red meat and poultry. For most finfish, the numbers are in the same range—around 45 to 75 milligrams of cholesterol per 3-ounce cooked portion. Some shellfish, namely shrimp (166 mg per 3 oz.) and calamari (248 mg per 3 oz.), is very high in dietary cholesterol. See the Seafood's Nutrition Assets and Liabilities chart on page 165 for more information.

Fish is low in sodium content which has another health benefit. To maintain this health benefit, low sodium preparation methods need to be used. The Seafood's Nutrition Assets and Liabilities chart on page 165 shows that a few items, such as surimi (imitation crab), blue crab, lobster, and shrimp, are slightly higher in sodium.

However, you can't just eat fish in any restaurant without carefully considering the meal. Most fast-food preparations of fish destroy anything healthy about it. Several fast-food seafood chains offer a few healthier baked and broiled items, but by and large, most of their seafood offerings are battered and fried.

Be adventurous with seafood. There are many varieties of finfish served in seafood and upscale restaurants. Consider monkfish, Chilean sea bass, mahi mahi or ahi tuna. There are also many delicious lowfat preparations available. Try poached salmon, steamed halibut with vegetables, barbecued shrimp, mesquite-grilled tuna, swordfish kebabs, braised monkfish with wine sauce, and blackened mahi mahi.

As your dining companions fill up on high-fat cups of New England clam chowder and fried calamari or shrimp, you can start with a healthy appetizer from the raw bar: oysters on the half shell, tuna tartare, yellowtail sashimi, mussels steeped in garlic wine sauce, shrimp cocktail, or ceviche. At the raw bar, almost all the items are very low in fat. Raw oysters, clams, and mussels are most often served with very low-calorie sauces, such as a tomato-based red cocktail sauce or a broth-based garlic sauce.

If you are planning to eat raw fish, make sure that the restaurant sells a lot of it. When it arrives, look at and smell the fish to make sure it is fresh. If you're in doubt, don't eat it. Read more about eating sushi and sashimi in Chapter 8 on Japanese food.

Surimi is the crabmeat lookalike that is substituted or used in combination with crabmeat for seafood salads and casseroles in moderately priced restaurants. Surimi is most often made from pollack, which actually gets good ratings for containing healthy fish oils and contains minimal mercury levels. Surimi is low in calories, fat, and cholesterol, but it is a bit higher in sodium than other finfish because it is processed. It also contains a bit of sugar, which contributes to its carbohydrate count. Surimi is much less expensive and more available than crabmeat, which is why it has gained popularity. If you spot a menu listing "seafood" salad, it will probably contain surimi. Even though surimi is basically healthy on its own, it can become high in fat very quickly when mixed with mayonnaise or topped with a cream sauce.

For your main course, you'll have to look carefully to avoid the fat. You'll see red flag words like "stuffed with," "covered in cream sauce," or "drawn butter" on most seafood menus that should be avoided. Instead, look for the green flag words that indicate lower-fat preparations.

Practice portion control from the starting gate. Consider sharing an entrée. Many entrées include as much as 8 to 10 ounces of fish. Split the portion with a dining companion or put half into a to-go container. If you're in a restaurant with a salad bar, split a fish entrée and visit the salad bar to round out your meal. Try a seafood dish served over pasta, such as shrimp linguini with stir-fry vegetables or fettuccine with white clam sauce. (Just make sure you don't end up with a thick cream or butter sauce.) Even a healthy preparation is probably enough for two. Grilled fish or crabcake sandwiches have moderate carbs and protein, but skip the dollop of tartar sauce slopped on top. Instead, ask for a side of cocktail sauce and use it like ketchup.

Seafood's Nutrition Assets and Liabilities

Food Item—Finfish	Calories	Grams of Fat	% Calories as Fat	Cholesterol	Sodium
Bluefish	135	5	33	65	65
Catfish	130	7	48	54	68
Cod (Scrod)	89	1	10	47	66
Flounder/Sole	99	1	9	58	89
Haddock	95	1	9	63	74
Halibut	119	3	23	35	59
Mackerel (Pacific)	171	9	47	51	94
Mahi Mahi (Dolphin Fish)	93	1	10	80	96
Monkfish	82	2	23	27	20
Pollack	100	1	9	77	94
Salmon (Sockeye)	184	9	44	74	56
Salmon (Atlantic)	175	11	57	54	52
Surimi (Imitation Crabmeat) (Note: High in sodium and contains 13 g carbohydrate)	81	0	0	25	715
Swordfish	132	4	27	42	98
Trout (Rainbow)	144	6	38	58	36
Tuna, Bluefin	156	5	29	42	42
Tuna, Light, Canned in Water (high in sodium)	99	1	9	26	297

Food Item—Shellfish	Calories	Grams of Fat	% Calories as Fat	Cholesterol	Sodium
Calamari (High in Cholesterol)	98	2	18	248	47
Crab, blue (High in Sodium)	87	2	21	85	237
Lobster (High in Sodium)	81	3	33	61	283
Shrimp (High in Cholesterol)	84	1	11	166	190

*All information is based on one 3-ounce cooked edible portion with no fat used in its preparation. Nutrition information is obtained from the USDA's National Nutrient Database for Standard Reference (http://www.ars.usda.gov/nutrientdata).

▷ Green Flag Words

Ingredients

△ all finfish and shellfish (raw and cooked)

△ all herbs, spices, garlic, and seasonings

△ wasabi

△ pickled ginger

△ vegetables (all types)

Cooking Methods/Menu Descriptions/Names

△ broiled

△ blackened

△ Cajun style

△ mesquite-grilled or grilled

△ marinated

△ barbecued

△ stir-fried (be aware of increased sodium)

△ teriyaki (be aware of increased sodium)

△ steamed

△ seared

△ kebabs

△ white or red clam sauce

△ served with tomato or fruit salsa

▶ Red Flag Words

Ingredients

▼ cheese

▼ drawn butter

▼ bread crumbs (usually means sautéed or fried)

▼ stuffing

▼ bacon, sausage

▼ coconut

Cooking Methods/Menu Descriptions/Names

▼ fried, deep-fried

▼ breaded and fried, battered and fried

▼ fish 'n' chips

▼ hush puppies

▼ cream or cheese sauce

▼ casserole

▼ lobster or seafood pie

▼ Newburg or thermidor

▼ creamy chowder or bisque

▼ coconut crusted

At the Table

▼ tartar sauce

▼ mayonnaise-based sauces

▼ rolls and butter

▼ oyster crackers

Special Requests

- "Please broil my seafood dry with a few bread crumbs."
- "Bring me a few extra lemon wedges."
- "May I get a side of cocktail sauce rather than tartar sauce?"
- "Please serve the salad with dressing on the side."
- "Do you have balsamic vinegar I could use on my salad?"
- "Could I substitute a baked potato for French fries?"
- "Could I substitute a dinner salad or steamed vegetable for the creamy coleslaw?"
- "Please bring the butter and sour cream on the side."
- "Could I get a to-go container at the beginning of my meal?"
- "Please bring an extra plate. We are going to share."
- "Please bring my appetizer as my main course, but I'll have my salad when they have their appetizers."

Typical Menu: Seafood Style

✲ *Indicates preferred choices*

Raw Bar

- ✲ **Oysters** on the halfshell
- ✲ **Cherrystone clams** on the halfshell
- ✲ **Assorted sashimi** served with wasabi, pickled ginger, and soy sauce
- ✲ **Raw bar assortment** (oysters, clams, crab claws, and shrimp)

Appetizers

- **Baked clams Casino**
- ✲ **Steamed clams**
- **Fried calamari** with spicy tomato sauce

- ☼ **Marinated calamari**
- ☼ **Mussels marinara**
- **Oysters Rockefeller**
- ☼ **Barbecued shrimp**
- ☼ **Crab cakes** (sautéed or fried) (Note: choose sautéed, consider as main course)
- **Shrimp tempura**
- ☼ **Shrimp cocktail**—6 large shrimp with cocktail sauce

Soups

- ☼ **Shrimp gumbo**
- ☼ **Fish chowder** (light fish-stock base with onions, carrots and leeks)
- **New England clam chowder**
- ☼ **Manhattan clam chowder**
- **Lobster bisque**

Broiled, Steamed, Grilled, or Blackened Fish

- ☼ **Bluefish**
- ☼ **Chilean sea bass**
- ☼ **Cod**
- ☼ **Halibut**
- ☼ **Mahi mahi** (dolphin fish)
- ☼ **Monkfish**
- ☼ **Salmon**
- ☼ **Swordfish**

Fried Fish

- **Bass**
- **Catfish**
- **Flounder**
- **Haddock**

Finfish Entrées

✿ **Broiled mackerel** with light mustard and dill sauce

Baked stuffed sole

Scrod, stuffed and baked, covered with cheese sauce

✿ **Swordfish kebabs** with peppers, mushrooms, and red onions

Shellfish Entrées

Baked stuffed jumbo shrimp

✿ **Steamed Maine lobster** (with drawn butter and lemon, served with corn on the cob, creamy coleslaw, and watermelon—skip the butter and the coleslaw)

Lobster pie (lobster meat in cream sauce casserole, topped with bread crumbs)

✿ **Scallops** (sautéed in a spicy tomato sauce)

✿ **Alaskan king crab claws** (steamed and served with drawn butter)

Seafood casserole (crabmeat, shrimp, scallops, and others combined with Parmesan cheese cream sauce and topped with bread crumbs)

✿ **Cioppino** (clams, shrimp, lobster, and calamari braised in tomato sauce and served over pasta)

✿ **Bouillabaisse** (seafood stew with monkfish, cod, and lobster)

Side Items

French fries

✿ **Baked potato**

✿ **Saffron rice**

✿ **Rice pilaf**

✿ **Tossed green salad**

Creamy coleslaw
❖ Sautéed zucchini
Yellow squash and onion
❖ Steamed fresh broccoli

Desserts

New York cheesecake
❖ Fresh strawberries or raspberries with crème de cassis and
whipped cream
Chocolate layer cake
Apple pie à la mode with vanilla ice cream

···················· ◀ "May I Take Your Order" ▶ ····················
Low-Calorie Sample Meal

Tossed green salad (dressing
on the side)
Quantity: 2 cups
Lemon-basil vinaigrette
dressing
Quantity: 1 tablespoon
Sautéed scallops (in spicy to-
mato sauce)
Quantity: 1½ cups
Saffron rice
Quantity: ⅔ cup
Broccoli, steamed fresh (hold butter)
Quantity: ½ cup

NUTRITION SUMMARY
540 calories
Carb: 51 g, 38%
Fat: 19 g, 31%
Protein: 42 g, 31%
Cholesterol: 60 mg
Sodium: 1100 mg

Moderate-Calorie Sample Meal

Fish chowder (½ order)
Quantity: ½ cup
Steamed clams (with lemon
and clam broth)
Quantity: 10 to 15 clams
Steamed Maine lobster (with
drawn butter and lemon—
hold the butter)
Quantity: 1½-lb lobster
Corn on the cob (hold the butter and salt)
Quantity: 2 ears
Watermelon
Quantity: 2 cups

> **NUTRITION SUMMARY**
> 715 calories
> Carb: 73 g, 41%
> Fat: 25 g, 31%
> Protein: 52 g, 29%
> Cholesterol: 165 mg
> Sodium: 1350 mg

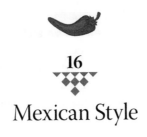

16

Mexican Style

Mexican food is among America's top three favorite cuisines, and it's available pretty much anywhere—from California to Maine. Variety abounds: Mexican eateries range from independent, authentic, and even upscale sit-down restaurants to more typical moderately priced sit-down chains which are all promoting the freshness of their food, such as Chevy's, Chi-Chi's, and Pepe's. Taco Bell leads the pack in the fast-food Mexican restaurant category, but there's also Del Taco and Taco John's. A new breed of fast-casual Mexican chains, such as Baja Fresh, Chipotle Mexican Grill, Qdoba Mexican Grill, and Rubio's has emerged. In several of these chains, customers pick their own "fixings." This is great for healthy eating—you can pile on the healthy items and skip the unhealthy ones.

Most Mexican dishes highlight five ingredients: rice, corn, beans, tomatoes, and chilies. The good news is they're healthy—high in vitamins and minerals and low in fat. Meat—often ground or shredded beef, pork, or chicken—is served in small portions, which minimizes saturated fat and cholesterol. Spicy toppings—red or green salsa, pico de gallo, and chilies—up the vegetable count and add great flavor with next to no calories.

Don't get carried away, though. The health attributes of the key ingredients can be trumped if foods are fried, refried, or smothered with cheese or sour cream, as they often are in dishes such as loaded nachos, chimichangas, and Mexican salads served in a fried tortilla bowl. Don't despair: Some Mexican meals are healthy. Soft tacos filled with refried beans, lettuce, tomato, onions, and salsa; chicken enchiladas; fajitas; and fresh salads are just a few of the healthier dishes you can choose.

Nutrition Snapshot

The following nutrition snapshot is intended to provide you with the nutrition numbers for a handful of common menu items served at Mexican restaurants. You'll see nutrition data that ranges from mind-blowing to healthy. Use them to educate yourself about the nutrition facts of your current Mexican foods. If necessary, make changes to eat healthier.

Menu Item	Calories	Carbohydrate (g)	Fat (g)	Saturated Fat (g)	*Trans* Fat (g)	Sodium (mg)
Tortilla Chips—2 oz (Qdoba)	290	38	14	2	0	170
Send them away or just take a handful, but don't resist the salsa. It's nearly no-cal with lots of zip. Use it as a salad dressing or as a topping for other dishes.						
Nachos—Macho (Del Taco)	1100	113	63	24	na	2640
Most people wouldn't order this to eat alone, but don't even think about sharing this either.						
Refried Beans (Refritos)—1 serving (Taco John's)	395	50	15	5	4	1110
Look for cooked black or pinto beans instead.						
Breakfast Quesadilla (Sausage)— 1 (Taco John's)	735	42	45	22	1	1500
Skip it. This contains as much fat as you should eat in an entire day.						
Chili Cheese Fries (Del Taco)	670	51	46	na	15	880
Skip 'em. They're a nutritional disaster.						

Menu Item	Calories	Carbohydrate (g)	Fat (g)	Saturated Fat (g)	*Trans* Fat (g)	Sodium (mg)
Soft Chicken Taco (Del Taco)	210	16	12	na	4	520
Reasonable choice—order with Mexican rice and salad. Top with tasty salsa or pico de gallo.						
Chicken Fajita without Tortillas and with Tamalito, Rice, Sour Cream and Guacamole (Chevy's)	913	67	45	16	na	1757 (tamalito sauce adds ~ 600 mg sodium)
Fajitas are often one of the healthier Mexican picks. However, skip the sour cream and the guacamole and don't go it alone—split or make two meals.						
Spicy Jack Chicken Quesadilla (Del Taco)	570	40	30	18	na	1300
Wow! The cheese really runs up the fat count.						
Mahi Mahi Ensalada (Baja Fresh)	280	20	9	3	na	1010
A healthy choice.						
Cheese Enchilada—1 (Rubio's)	360	24	21	12	na	540
A reasonable choice if you've got the fat and saturated fat grams to spare. Pair it with a salad to fill you up.						
Seven-Layer Burrito—1 (Taco Bell)	490	25	18	7	1	1350
Skip it. You've got healthier options.						
Gordita—Supreme Steak—1 (Taco Bell)	290	28	13	5	0	530
A reasonable choice.						
Bean Burrito—1 (Taco John's)	380	53	10	5	2	830
A reasonable choice.						
Crunchy Chicken Taco Salad without Dressing (Taco Bell)	710	56	40	10	0	1070
Crunchy is a word to disguise "fried." Supreme is a word to disguise a large size or lots of high-fat toppings. A soft taco is a healthier choice.						

The Menu Profile

At most sit-down Mexican restaurants, you receive chips and salsa without asking for them. Before you know it, the basket's empty and is quickly refilled. The tortilla chips are deep-fried and heavily salted (to boost your orders of number of margaritas or beers). Exercise willpower and promise yourself to limit the number of chips you eat, or better yet, never let the basket land on the table.

Salsa is the winning half of the partnership. Red or green salsa is made with tomatoes, onions, garlic, chilies, cilantro, and salt. It has almost no fat and very few calories. Better yet, it makes a topping with plenty of pizzazz. Use salsa on salads or entrées in lieu of salad dressing, sour cream, and guacamole. Pico de gallo, which is often found on Mexican menus, is chopped tomatoes and onions and can be used as a substitute for salsa.

Appetizers offer a few healthy choices, but there are also many high-fat, fried items. The healthier choices are gazpacho, ceviche, chili con carne, and tortilla or black bean soup. The appetizers to avoid or limit are nachos, super nachos, chili con queso, quesadillas, and guacamole and chips. If your dining companions order high-fat appetizers, start with a cup of chili, black bean soup, or a dinner salad.

Mexican cuisine has a much lighter dependence on meats than American fare. Compare the small quantity of meat, one to two ounces, in one enchilada to an 8- to 10-ounce steak.

Unfortunately, fat is the biggest villain in Mexican cuisine. There are many fried items, and many Mexican recipes traditionally call for the use of lard or other animal-fat products, which contain significant amounts of cholesterol and saturated fat. However, as large restaurant chains are facing significant pressure about using shortenings, more and more are using healthier liquid oils.

When you place your order, ask your server if the restaurant uses 100 percent liquid vegetable oil or less healthy vegetable shortening, beef tallow, or lard. Knowing that a taco shell will be fried in an unhealthy shortening may prompt you to order a soft enchilada instead. If vegetable oil is used for food preparation, you can feel better about ordering chicken or beef fajitas. If calories are your biggest concern, limit fat any way you can.

Mexican food can also be high in sodium. Salt is used in many recipes, and a lot of the food-prep work is done in advance, such as spicing meats to stuff into tacos or burritos. This makes it difficult to request that salt be omitted. However, when you order a dish featuring grilled chicken, fish, or beef in an upscale Mexican restaurant, you may be successful with a hold-the-salt request. Chips, salsa, and large amounts of cheese can also contribute to raising the sodium level. Green or red salsa can be used to add punch to salads or chicken and fish dishes instead, and it is fine to use in small amounts.

Mexican entrées frequently contain chicken, beans, corn- or wheat-based "breads," lettuce, tomatoes, onions, and chilies. All are healthy ingredients. Keep them in mind as you decide what to order. Many high-fat and high-calorie ingredients are also found in Mexican entrées, such as cheese, sour cream, and chorizo (Mexican sausage). Chicken or beef enchiladas, burritos, or soft tacos are great choices. Fajitas are a healthy choice, and you can choose from chicken, shrimp, beef, or a combination. One order often is enough for two. Request extra tortillas.

A bowl of chili con carne (hold the cheese, but load on the onions) is a good choice to pair with a side salad. A Mexican main-course salad with either spicy chicken or beef is another healthy alternative, but be sure to ask that your salad be served in a dish rather than a tortilla shell. Some upscale Mexican restaurants offer a grilled chicken or fish dish served with a spicy tomato sauce, which is a particularly healthy choice. It's always smart to ask that the high-fat add-ons be left off the order or served "on the side," such as sour cream, guacamole, cheese, and olives.

Along with Mexican dinners come the starches: usually Mexican rice and refried beans. Beans, which may be pinto, kidney, or black, are high in complex carbohydrates and have considerable cholesterol-lowering soluble fiber, but if they're fried in lard, you should stay away. It's a better idea to skip the refritos and order a side of unfried black beans, Mexican rice, or soft tortillas.

If you want to pick and choose exactly what you want, order à la carte. If you are watching your calories and fat intake, a single chicken enchilada or a bean burrito paired with a dinner salad will enable you to avoid the high-fat accompaniments. Steer clear of combination plates unless you plan to share, as they typically have far too much food and include many high-fat items.

The list of desserts in Mexican restaurants is minimal. A typical Mexican dessert is the high-fat, high-sugar disaster sopapilla, which is deep-fried dough. Flan, an egg custard with caramel topping, is another familiar Mexican dessert. It's not a terrible choice, but it should be avoided if you are watching your cholesterol. You can always opt for a flavorful cup of black Mexican coffee instead in upscale restaurants.

▷ Green Flag Words

Ingredients

△ shredded spicy chicken, beef, or ground beef

△ lettuce, tomatoes, onions

△ chilies

△ black beans, pinto beans

△ salsa, green or red

△ enchilada sauce

△ mole sauce

△ soft tortilla (corn or flour)

△ avocado

Cooking Methods/Menu Descriptions/Names

△ pico de gallo

△ wrapped in a soft tortilla

△ fajitas (best to share)

△ grilled

△ marinated

△ simmered

△ served with spicy tomato sauce

△ soft tacos

△ burritos

△ tostadas

△ arroz con pollo

△ tamales

△ guacamole

▶ Red Flag Words

Ingredients

▼ black olives

▼ sour cream

▼ cheese (any style: topped, stuffed, covered, shredded)

▼ chorizo (Mexican sausage)

▼ bacon

Cooking Methods/Menu Descriptions/Names

▼ cheese sauce

▼ cream sauce

▼ served in a tortilla shell

▼ served over tortilla or nacho chips
▼ crispy
▼ fried or deep-fried
▼ layered with refried beans
▼ chili con queso
▼ nachos with cheese
▼ cheese quesadillas
▼ chimichangas
▼ tacos

At the Table

▼ tortilla chips
▼ sour cream

Special Requests

- "Please hold (or serve on the side) the sour cream or guacamole." (Note: If you can afford the calories, guacamole has health attributes.)
- "Please serve my salad without the fried tortilla shell (or nacho chips) but bring an à la carte order of soft tortillas."
- "Please take the chips away from the table, but I'll use the salsa on my food."
- "Please don't bring any chips to the table, but do bring the salsa."
- "Please hold the cheese."
- "Would it be possible to get extra salsa, green or red sauce, and pico de gallo (near-zero-calorie sauces) on the side?"
- "Please put extra shredded lettuce, tomatoes, and chopped onions on the plate."

- "Would it be possible to substitute shredded chicken for the beef?"
- "We will share the fajitas. Can you bring a few extra tortillas?"
- "May I have black beans instead of refried beans?"
- "Could I get this wrapped up to take home?"

Typical Menu: Mexican-Style

✿ *Indicates preferred choices*

Appetizers

Tostada chips (with salsa)
Tostada chips (with guacamole)
Nachos (with melted cheese and jalapeño peppers)
Chili con queso (melted cheese, green chilies, and peppers with corn tortilla chips)
✿ **Black bean soup** (cup or bowl)
✿ **Chili con carne** (cup or bowl)
✿ **Gazpacho** (spicy cold soup made from vegetables and tomatoes)

Salads

Tell your server to hold the sour cream and the fried tortilla shell. Ask for dressing to be served on the side.

✿ **Dinner salad** (mixed greens, cheese, and tomato, topped with onions)
Mexican salad (lettuce, tomato, and bell peppers, topped with two kinds of cheese, served in crisp tortilla shell with creamy garlic dressing)
✿ **Taco salad** (choice of spicy ground meat or shredded chicken, topped with refried beans, lettuce, tomatoes, and

onions, topped with sour cream and guacamole and served in crisp tortilla shell)

✿ **Tostada salad** (choice of spicy strips of beef or chicken topped with refried beans, lettuce, tomatoes, and onions, topped with sour cream and guacamole and served on a warm tostada)

Mexican Specialties

Tell your server to serve the sour cream, guacamole, and cheese on the side. Consider splitting a meal—particularly fajitas—with a dining companion.

Chimichangas, beef or chicken (flour tortillas filled with spicy beef or chicken and Monterey Jack cheese, fried, and topped with tomato sauce)

✿ **Fajitas** (marinated beef, chicken, or shrimp grilled with onions, green peppers, lettuce, diced tomatoes, sour cream, and guacamole)

✿ **Enchiladas** (corn tortillas stuffed with either ground beef or shredded chicken and topped with tomato sauce, shredded cheese, and sour cream)

Tacos (hard) (fried flour or corn tortillas stuffed with choice of spicy ground beef, shredded chicken, or a seafood blend; loaded with shredded lettuce, diced tomatoes, and onions and topped with cheese)

✿ **Tacos (soft)** (soft flour or corn tortillas stuffed with choice of spicy ground beef, shredded chicken, or a seafood blend; loaded with shredded lettuce, diced tomatoes, and onions and topped with cheese)

✿ **Burritos** (large flour tortillas filled with choice of refried beans and cheese, vegetables, spicy ground beef, or chicken;

served with tomato sauce and topped with shredded cheese)

Mexican Dinners

Served with refried beans and Mexican rice.

Flautas con crema (crisp rolled tortillas stuffed with shredded chicken or beef and topped with a spicy cream sauce)
✡ **Chili verde** (pork simmered with green chilies, vegetables, and Mexican spices)
✡ **Mole pollo** (boned chicken breast cooked in a hot and spicy mole sauce,)
✡ **Camarones de hacha** (fresh shrimp sautéed in a red- and green-tomato coriander sauce)
Carne asada (grilled sirloin steak served in an enchilada sauce with chorizo and guacamole)
✡ **Arroz con pollo** (boneless chicken breast served on top of spicy rice with vegetable sauce)

Side Orders

✡ **Mexican rice**
Refried beans
✡ **Black beans**
✡ **Tortillas, flour or corn**
✡ **Pico de gallo**
✡ **Guacamole**

Desserts

✡ **Flan** (caramel-flavored custard)
Sopapillas (deep-fried dough, tossed in sugar)

·············· ◀ **"May I Take Your Order?"** ▶ ···············

Low-Calorie Sample Meal

Chili con carne
Quantity: 1 cup
Dinner salad (hold the cheese and dressing)
Quantity: 2 cups
Salsa for dressing
Chicken taco, soft
Quantity: 1

NUTRITION SUMMARY
480 calories
Carb: 47 g, 39%
Fat: 20 g, 35%
Protein: 31 g, 26%
Cholesterol: 67 mg
Sodium: 1600 mg

Moderate-Calorie Sample Meal

Black bean soup
Quantity: 1 cup
Chili verde served with 2 flour tortillas
Quantity: 1½ cups
Mexican rice
Quantity: 1½ cups
Refried beans
Quantity: ⅓ cup
Mexican beer
Quantity: 12 oz.

NUTRITION SUMMARY
990 calories
Carb: 118 g, 48%
Fat: 30 g, 27%
Protein: 42 g, 17%
Alcohol: 8%
Cholesterol: 96 mg
Sodium: 2100 mg

Mexican Menu Lingo

Arroz: The Spanish word for rice. Mexican rice is long-grain white rice with sautéed tomatoes, onions, and garlic added for flavor.

Burrito: a soft wheat-flour tortilla filled with chicken, beef, cheese and/or beans, rice, salsa, cheese, and sour cream. Some restaurants have begun to serve tortilla-free burritos.

Carne: the Spanish word for meat.

Cerveza: the Spanish word for beer.

Ceviche: raw seafood (usually shrimp or scallops) marinated or "cooked" in lime or lemon juice for many hours and served as an appetizer or light meal.

Chilies: there are over 100 different types of chilies native to Mexico. They are of different shapes, sizes, and colors, and they vary in level of spiciness from mild to hot. Chilies are available fresh, pickled, and dried.

Chili con carne: usually simply called "chili" in America, a thick soup made with tomatoes, onions, peppers, beans, and chilies for a kick. Con carne means "with meat," which may be ground, shredded, or in chunks. Vegetarian chili contains no meat. Chili con carne is often served with raw chopped onions and shredded cheese.

Chimichanga: a deep-fried flour tortilla filled with beef, chicken, cheese, and/or beans and served with a tomato-based sauce.

Chorizo: a hot and highly seasoned Mexican pork sausage.

Cilantro: a leafy green herb with a distinctive flavor frequently used in Mexican cooking; also called coriander.

Enchiladas: corn tortillas dipped in enchilada sauce, warmed on a flat grill with small amount of oil, and filled with a choice of chicken, beef, or cheese; served topped with light tomato-based enchilada sauce.

Fajitas: sautéed chicken or beef served with sautéed onions and green peppers, shredded lettuce, tomatoes, guacamole and sour cream; served with flour or corn tortillas. Usually you roll your own at the table and there's usually enough for two.

Flan: a baked custard with a caramel topping; contains mainly sugar, eggs, and cream and whole or condensed milk.

Gazpacho: a spicy, cold, tomato-based soup containing puréed or chopped tomatoes, cucumbers, peppers, and onions.

Guacamole: a spread made of mashed avocado, onion, tomatoes, garlic, lemon juice, and spices that is served as a topping, as a dip with chips, or on the side. Avocado is high in fat, with approximately 80 calories per ¼ avocado, but the fat is mainly monounsaturated and contains no cholesterol.

Jalapeño chili: a very small, hot, green chili often mistakenly referred to as a pepper. Used to spice or top certain menu items.

Mole: a spicy brown seasoning mixture or sauce that is used on chicken or other meats; it contains a small amount of chocolate.

Quesadillas: flour tortillas filled with a cheese and chili mixture (and sometimes a meat filling), rolled, and then fried.

Refried beans: pinto beans that have been cooked, fried in lard, and seasoned with onions, garlic, and chilies.

Salsa: a hot red sauce made from tomatoes, onions, and chilies, it appears on the tables of most Mexican restaurants.

Salsa verde: a very hot green sauce made from tomatillos, which are Mexican green tomatoes, and other spices.

Taco: a corn tortilla filled with meat or chicken, shredded cheese, lettuce, and tomatoes; usually the corn tortilla is fried in the shape of a "U." Soft tacos are usually made with a flour tortilla and are not fried.

Tamale: a spicy filling of either meat or chicken, surrounded by moist cornmeal dough and wrapped in corn husks or banana leaves. They are steamed.

Tortilla: the "bread" of Mexico, a very thin circle of dough made either from corn or flour; corn tortillas are also fried to make taco shells or chips.

Tostadas: crisp, deep-fried tortilla chips, or the whole fried tortilla, which are then covered with various toppings, including cheese, beans, lettuce, tomato, and/or onions.

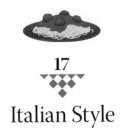

17

Italian Style

Americans love Italian food. You can eat healthfully—a cup of minestrone or stracciatelle (Italy's answer to egg-drop soup), linguine with white clam sauce, and a demitasse of espresso makes a delicious and sensible meal. But at the opposite end of the spectrum, you can order meals loaded with fat, cholesterol, and sodium: garlic bread doused in butter; an antipasto platter of Italian cheeses, Genoa salami, marinated artichokes, and olives; an entrée portion of fettuccine Alfredo; and a cannoli for dessert. A wide range of choices—from healthier to not-so-healthy—awaits you at Italian restaurants and portion control will always be the skill to use to prevent overeating.

Today, you can eat Italian food in a wide array of settings, from inexpensive eateries in airports or food courts to elegant bistros and four-star restaurants. Italian food is served in thousands of independent restaurants from coast to coast. A growing list of national sit-down restaurant chains, such as Buca di Beppo, Carrabba's Italian Grill, Fazoli's, Maggiano's Little Italy, Olive Garden, and Romano's Macaroni Grill, serve bottomless bowls of pasta. Pizza Hut, California Pizza Kitchen, and Sbarro split their menus between popular Italian entrées and pizza. Pizza is one of the most common choices for American families when dining out or ordering in. It is a fast, convenient crowd-pleaser. Look for information on pizza in Chapter 18: Pizza Style.

Nutrition Snapshot

The following nutrition snapshot is intended to provide you with nutrition data for some common menu items served at Italian restaurants. You'll see nutrition data that ranges from mind-blowing to healthy. Use them to educate yourself about the nutrition makeup of your current Italian favorites. If necessary, make changes to eat healthier.

Menu Item	Calories	Carbohydrate (g)	Fat (g)	Saturated Fat (g)	*Trans* Fat (g)	Sodium (mg)
Garlic Bread Stick—1 (Fazoli's)	150	20	7	1.5	0	290
Stick with Italian bread dipped lightly in olive oil or marinara sauce (an even healthier choice).						
Minestrone Soup—1 serving (Fazoli's)	120	23	1	0	na	910
A healthy choice with hearty beans. Good filler.						
Penne with Marinara—small (Fazoli's)	450	88	3	0	0	770
A reasonable choice, but high in carbohydrate. Ask a dining companion to order a meat dish and split the two meals.						
Chicken Giardiano—entrée (Olive Garden)	560	59	15	3	na	1180
A reasonable choice, but high in sodium.						
Spaghetti with Sauce—dinner (Sbarro)	820	120	28	na	na	890
A healthy choice, but too much food. Order an appetizer size, split it, or take half of it home.						
Shrimp Primavera—entrée (Olive Garden)	706	84	18	4	na	1220
Perfect to split. Complement with a salad.						
Spaghetti with Chicken Parmesan— dinner (Sbarro)	930	75	36	na	na	950
Try a healthier option with a lower fat gram count.						
Ravioli with Meat Sauce—dinner (Fazoli's)	550	71	20	10	0	1460
A reasonable choice, but high in sodium.						

Menu Item	Calories	Carbohydrate (g)	Fat (g)	Saturated Fat (g)	*Trans* Fat (g)	Sodium (mg)
Pepperoni Stromboli –1 (Sbarro)	890	82	44	na	na	2470
The fat count is high, largely because of the pepperoni. Order a veggie stromboli instead and/or split it.						
Chicken Marsala—entrée (Olive Garden)	973	66	57	na	na	1399
Wow. More fat than a person should consume in a day.						
Meat Lasagna—dinner (Sbarro)	650	36	37	na	na	1130
High fat count. Split it with a dining companion.						
Spaghetti with Alfredo—regular (Fazoli's)	780	125	18	6	0	1600
For an Alfredo, the fat count is low, but the carbs and the sodium are high. Split if you've just got to have Alfredo, and order a salad.						

The Menu Profile

As the menu is placed in front of you, crusty Italian bread with butter or olive oil, garlic rolls, garlic bread, bread sticks, ciabbata bread, or focaccia (Italian flat bread) may end up on the table alongside it. Unadulterated whole-grain bread is your best bet, but it's rare in Italian restaurants. Other than the commonly served white Italian bread, most of the other breads are loaded with fat even before you spread butter on them or dip them in olive oil. If your calorie limits allow it, try one piece of bread and ask for a small dish of tomato (or marinara) sauce to dip it in. If you have even more calories to spare, dip your bread in olive oil instead of butter: olive oil contains "good fats" and no cholesterol. If it's hard to resist, ask the server to remove the bread.

If you are watching your calories, select a lowfat entrée and a green salad. If you have more calories and fat to "spend," consider an antipasto (appetizer) or broth-based soup. Healthy antipasto choices can be hard to find, but they are often available. Try squid, mussels, or clams prepared in a lemon-garlic-herb-wine (any combination) or tomato sauce. If you're not watching your sodium, you might consider an antipasto of marinated vegetables, such as peppers, pickles, and olives. You may choose low-calorie bruschetta (tomatoes, olive oil, and garlic brushed on slices of Italian bread) or sliced tomatoes served with fresh mozzarella (watch the mozzarella). Antipastos loaded with cheeses and Italian cold cuts are little more than pure fat, including saturated fat and cholesterol. Steer clear of anything deep-fried, including mozzarella, calamari, and zucchini sticks.

Of course, the cornerstone of Italian food is pasta. Pasta is made with flour, water, and sometimes eggs. It takes many different shapes and forms. Familiarize yourself with the varieties of pasta in the section "Know Your Pasta" at the end of this chapter. With no sauce or mixed ingredients, pasta contains no fat—it's just carbohydrates with a bit of protein. Unfortunately, most restaurants aren't yet serving the whole-grain or whole-wheat pasta that is now available in grocery stores. Keep searching for it on menus, however—it is a healthier choice because of its high fiber content.

Arguably the greatest challenge with eating pasta in restaurants is the huge portions. Your portion control weaponry? Split an order, put half the order in a take-home box immediately after it arrives on the table, or order an appetizer-size serving.

Try the flavored pastas: spinach, squid ink, or tomato. The added flavor will help you savor your dining experience and will make you feel more satisfied—without adding a significant amount of calories.

Those calories can add up fast, however, depending on what your pasta is topped or stuffed with. Is the sauce tomato-based and loaded with onions and garlic (such as a marinara sauce), or is it loaded with high-fat ingredients like cheeses, sausage, cream, and/or bacon (such as a carbonara sauce). Your challenge is to include the green flag words in your order and limit the red flag words.

Don't worry. You can always find healthy pasta choices. Look for marinara, primavera (sautéed vegetables), red or white clam sauce, or bolognese. Avoid the "stuffed" pastas, such as ravioli, cannelloni, and manicotti, because they are usually stuffed with cheese alone or other ingredients combined with cheese or butter. You can consider a stuffed pasta if it's stuffed with vegetables, but ask for details before you proceed—it may be topped with a cream sauce. If you are carefully watching your calories and fat, pesto should be avoided. It's made with basil, that's a good start, but three high-fat ingredients are usually in the mix as well: pignoli (pine) nuts, olive oil, and Parmesan cheese. Just because it's green doesn't mean it's healthy. If you've got a few extra calories and fat grams to spend, a bit of pesto goes a long way.

Two other Italian taste treats found more commonly in upscale Italian restaurants are risotto and polenta, two grain-based dishes native to Italy. Risotto is made with Arborio rice, a short-grain rice with stubby kernels. It traces its ancestry to the Po Valley region of Italy, where it is grown in abundance. Unfortunately, chefs typically prepare risotto with lots of butter, cheese, sausage, and other high-fat ingredients. The taste might be great, but the fat, calories, and cholesterol will be high. If you want to try it, consider a meatless risotto that blends spices, herbs, and vegetables—risotto with spinach and mushrooms or risotto primavera.

Polenta is like cornmeal pudding. It is made with cornmeal, water, and salt and is a staple in the Veneto region of Italy. It is often served with sauces, many of which may load on the fat.

Some menus include triangles of polenta that have been grilled, which are a lowfat choice.

Insalata, or crunchy greens, are filling and low in calories—depending on what's sitting on top of them. Look for salads made with radicchio (red leaves), arugula (a strong-tasting green), endive, tomatoes, broccoli, mixed baby field greens, spinach, beets, peppers, onions, and other raw or marinated vegetables. A few olives or condiments like sun-dried tomatoes aren't a problem, but some Italian salads are loaded with extremely high-fat items like cheese, pasta salad, prosciutto (Italian ham), bacon, pancetta (Italian cured bacon), or nuts.

Order your dressing on the side, and look for a light one. Better yet, try a bit of olive oil with vinegar or a few fresh lemon wedges. Some of the newer Italian restaurants use flavored vinegars, such as tarragon or rosemary. If you spot it on the menu, you know it's in the kitchen. Ask for vinegar on the side to use alone or to stretch the dressing you've ordered. Avoid Caesar salad, which has a thick, heavy dressing and egg, grated cheese, and anchovies.

For your secondo piatto, or main course, you might find pollo, pesce, or carne, which are poultry, seafood, or meat, in that order. If you're having pasta, don't feel compelled to order a main course as well, unless you split it or take half home. It's simply too much protein (meat). If you do want a main course, select one of the grilled fish, scallops, or chicken breast choices. Always ask how the dish is prepared. Look for tomato-based or vegetable sauces or mushroom or wine sauces prepared without cream. It's common to see different meats prepared with the same sauces. Avoid the high-fat and high-sodium options, such as prosciutto (ham), pancetta (bacon), cheese, and cream sauces.

A popular Italian entrée is veal. Misconceptions about veal

exist. Many people believe that veal is relatively low in calories, fat, and cholesterol. Veal cutlet, which is the lean cut that is often used in Italian restaurants, is low in calories (about 40–50 per ounce cooked), but its cholesterol content is similar to that of lean beef (about 20–25 milligrams per ounce cooked). On the other side of the veal spectrum is veal breast, which is higher in fat (about 60–70 calories per ounce cooked). Unfortunately, many veal preparations of all cuts involve breading and sautéing, which adds extra calories and fat. If you have a few extra calories to spare, veal marsala, cacciatore, or piccata are acceptable choices. If calories are tight, choose grilled fish or chicken instead.

If you are offered a side dish of pasta with a choice of sauce, choose tomato sauce (marinara) or garlic and oil. Consider ordering your pasta plain and top it with a little of the sauce from your entrée.

For dessert, Italian menus list items such as spumoni, cannoli, tortoni, Italian ices, and fresh berries with liqueur and whipped cream. Think about splitting a dessert or choose the lower-fat Italian ices, sorbettos (sorbets), or fresh berries. Another option: End your meal as many do in Italy, with a demitasse of black espresso.

The Lowdown on Olives and Olive Oil

In central and south Italy, olive oil replaces butter as the fat of choice in recipes. That's a good thing, because monounsaturated fats and polyunsaturated fats are touted for their health value. Monounsaturated fats help lower LDLs (bad cholesterol) without decreasing HDLs (good cholesterol). Fatty ingredients that contain mainly monounsaturated fats, such as olive, canola, and peanut oils and nuts and avocados, have the added benefit of being cholesterol-free. For these reasons, olive oil is a healthy liquid oil to use at home and away. However, do remember that olive oil contains the same number of calories (50 calories per teaspoon) as every other fat, from butter to lard to hard vegetable shortening. As for olives, try all the varieties on salads, in Italian sauces, or just as a tasty side item, but remember that they are high in sodium and fat.

▷ Green Flag Words

Ingredients

△ onions, peppers, mushrooms

△ artichoke hearts (not marinated in oil)

△ sun-dried tomatoes

△ capers

△ spinach and other greens

△ marinated vegetables (not in oil)

△ grilled chicken, fish, seafood

△ herbs—basil and oregano

△ tomatoes (raw or cooked)

△ pasta—all types other than those stuffed with cheese and/or butter

△ olives, olive oil

Cooking Methods/Menu Descriptions/Names

△ lightly sautéed with onions and shallots

△ tomato-based sauces—marinara, bolognese, cacciatore, pomodoro, and puttanesca

△ tomato sauce and meatballs

△ white or red clam sauce

△ light red- or white-wine sauce

△ light mushroom and wine sauce

△ primavera (without cream)

△ piccata (a lemon sauce)

▶ Red Flag Words

Ingredients

- ▼ eggplant or zucchini (if fried)
- ▼ pancetta, prosciutto, or bacon
- ▼ sausage, veal, or pork
- ▼ butter
- ▼ cheese—mozzarella, Gorgonzola, Parmesan, provolone
- ▼ Italian cold cuts

Cooking Methods/Menu Descriptions/Names

- ▼ Alfredo
- ▼ carbonara
- ▼ saltimbocca
- ▼ parmigiana—veal, chicken, and eggplant
- ▼ stuffed with cheese
- ▼ creamy sauces—wine, mushroom, and cheese
- ▼ fried or deep-fried
- ▼ manicotti
- ▼ lasagna
- ▼ cannelloni
- ▼ stuffed shells

At the Table

- ▼ butter
- ▼ salad dressing
- ▼ grated cheese

Special Requests

- ◆ "Please don't bring us any bread."
- ◆ "Please take the olive oil (or butter) away."
- ◆ "Could I get a small amount of marinara sauce (or light tomato sauce) to dip the bread into?"

- "Please hold the Parmesan (or grated) cheese, bacon, olives, and pine nuts."
- "We are going to share a few items. Can these be split in the kitchen?"
- "Please put marinara sauce on my pasta, not olive oil."
- "Please use only a small amount of sauce over the pasta."
- "I'd like the appetizer-size pasta, and please bring it when you bring the other entrées."
- "Please remove my plate. I'm finished now."
- "I'll take the rest of this home."

Typical Menu: Italian Style

✡ *Indicates preferred choices*

Antipasto

Antipasto for two (marinated mushrooms, artichoke hearts, Genoa salami, pecorino, cheese)

Crispy zucchini sticks (fresh strips of zucchini and quick fried, served with marinara sauce)

✡ **Bruschetta** (fresh ripe tomatoes blended with garlic and balsamic vinegar on top of slices of Italian bread)

Prosciutto (wrapped around melon)

✡ **Marinated calamari**

Garlic bread

✡ **Marinated mushrooms**

✡ **Clams steamed in white wine**

Fried mozzarella sticks (with marinara sauce)

Zuppa (Soup)

✡ **Tortellini in broth**

✡ **Pasta e fagioli** (bean and pasta soup)

✡ **Minestrone**

Lentil and sausage
☼ **Stracciatelle** (a broth-based Italian chicken soup with semolina and spinach)

Insalata (Salad)

☼ **Arugula and Belgian endive** (with balsamic vinaigrette dressing)
☼ **Insalata, frutte di mare** (marinated seafood, scallops, shrimp, and calamari in a light marinade served on a bed of greens)
☼ **Insalata di casa** (house salad with greens, tomato, and onion)
Caesar salad (greens with buttery croutons, Parmesan cheese, and creamy Caesar dressing)
☼ **Spinach salad** (baby spinach leaves tossed with roasted red peppers and caramelized onions and topped with toasted pine nuts)

Pasta

Cannelloni (stuffed with ricotta cheese and spinach and topped with a light tomato sauce)
Ziti Bolognese (tubular noodles topped with a light tomato sauce containing ground meat, celery, carrots, and onions)
Linguine with pesto (flat pasta coated with traditional pesto)
Fettuccine Alfredo (a thin, flat pasta served with a creamy cheese sauce)
☼ **Angel hair pasta** (with white or red clam sauce)
☼ **Fusilli primavera** (a spiral-shaped pasta topped with a blend of spicy sautéed seasonal vegetables)

Carne (meat)

These entrées are generally served with a side of spaghetti that is topped with your choice of marinara sauce or olive oil and garlic.

Veal piccata (medallions of veal lightly sautéed in a butter, lemon, and wine sauce)

Veal cacciatore (a veal cutlet topped with tomato sauce, sautéed onions, mushrooms, and peppers)

Veal saltimbocca (cutlets breaded and sautéed and topped with prosciutto and provolone cheese)

❖ **Filet mignon** (an 8-ounce prime filet, broiled and finished with garlic butter; ask the server to hold the butter)

Pollo (Chicken)

These entrées are generally served with a side of spaghetti that is topped with your choice of marinara sauce or olive oil and garlic.

❖ **Chicken primavera** (a breast of chicken lightly sautéed and topped with sautéed seasonal vegetables)

Chicken parmigiana (a chicken cutlet baked with mozzarella cheese and tomato sauce)

Chicken in wine sauce (sautéed breast of chicken, roasted peppers, and mushrooms with Burgundy wine, fresh garlic, and rosemary)

Chicken marsala (chicken breasts sautéed with marsala wine, mushrooms, peas, and onions)

Pesce (Fish)

These entrées are generally served with a side of spaghetti that is topped with your choice of marinara sauce or olive oil and garlic.

☼ **Shrimp primavera** (sautéed shrimp and garden vegetables served on bed of angel-hair pasta)

☼ **Shrimp marinara** (shrimp lightly sautéed in garlic and topped with tomato sauce)

Scallops marsala (scallops sautéed with marsala wine, mushrooms, peas, and onions)

Shrimp scampi (shrimp sautéed in olive oil, fresh garlic, white wine, lemon, and oregano)

☼ **Sole primavera** (fillet of sole sautéed with an assortment of seasonal fresh vegetables, zucchini, peppers, and tomatoes)

Dolce

Tiramisu (espresso-soaked ladyfingers layered with custard and topped with cocoa)

Cheesecake (a rich cream cheese mixture atop a graham cracker crumb crust and topped with a berry sauce)

Spumoni (three flavors of ice cream topped with a fruity sauce)

Cannoli (a tube-shaped shell of pastry dough filled with a sweet creamy ricotta cheese)

☼ **Italian ice**

·················· ◀ **"May I Take Your Order"** ▶ ··················

Low-Calorie Sample Meal

Arugula and Belgian endive salad (request balsamic vinegar on the side)
Quantity: 2 cups
Shrimp primavera
(½ portion)
Quantity: 1½ cups
Espresso
Quantity: 1 cup

> **NUTRITION SUMMARY**
> 550 calories
> Carb: 62 g, 45%
> Fat: 21 g, 35% calories as fat
> Protein: 28 g, 20%
> Cholesterol: 160 mg
> Sodium: 650 mg

Moderate-Calorie Sample Meal

Tortellini (in broth)
Quantity: 1 cup
Insalata di casa (dressing on the side)
Quantity: 1 cup
Basil vinaigrette dressing
(on the side)
Quantity: 1 tablespoon
Veal cacciatore
Quantity: ½ order
Spaghetti (hold the sauce; use the sauce from the entrée instead)
Quantity: 1 cup

> **NUTRITION SUMMARY**
> 770 calories
> Carb: 87 g, 45%
> Fat: 21 g, 31%
> Protein: 46 g, 24%
> Cholesterol: 100 mg
> Sodium: 1050 mg

Know Your Pasta

Pasta, an Italian word meaning "paste" or "dough," is found on the menu of every Italian restaurant. Pasta is made of flour (durum, semolina, or all-purpose), water, and sometimes eggs. These ingredients are used to create a wide variety of different shapes, from angel hair to ziti. Today, there are also many different-colored pastas available: whole-wheat, whole-grain, tomato, spinach, artichoke, and more. This pasta primer will help you "Know Your Pasta" and have an easier time figuring out which are healthy and which aren't.

Agnolotti: crescent-shaped pieces of pasta stuffed with one or a combination of ingredients, such as cheese, meat, and spinach.

Angel hair: the thinnest and finest of the "long" pasta family, it is quite light in consistency and served with light, vegetable-based sauces.

Cannelloni: a large, tubular pasta similar to manicotti that is stuffed with one or a combination of ingredients, such as cheese, meat, and spinach.

Capellitti: Italian for "little hats," these are small stuffed pastas that look like little tortellinis. They are often stuffed with cheese or meats.

Fettuccine: a flat, long noodle about 1 inch wide, which is wider than linguine.

Fusilli: a spiral-shaped long pasta.

Gnocchi: little dumplings in ½-inch pieces made from flour, potatoes, or a combination of the two.

Lasagna: the widest noodle of the long, flat pastas, it is found with either smooth or scalloped edges.

Linguine: a flat, long noodle about ⅛-inch wide, which is thinner than fettuccine.

Manicotti: a long, tubular noodle about 2 inches in diameter that is most often stuffed with cheese and/or meat and served with tomato sauce.

Mostaccioli: a short, tubular noodle about 1½ inches long.

Penne: a short, tubular noodle that is quite similar to mostaccioli and rigatoni.

Ravioli: two pieces of pasta with a pocket in the middle. Traditionally, ravioli come in 2-inch squares, but smaller and round shapes are now available. Ravioli are always stuffed, traditionally with cheese, spinach, and/or meats. Today, you can find just about anything stuffed in ravioli, from butternut squash to duck confit.

Rigatoni: a short, tubular noodle quite similar to penne and mostaccioli.

Shells: noodles formed in the shape of conch shells. They are called conchiglie in Italian and found in a variety of sizes. Larger ones are stuffed, and most are served topped with tomato sauce.

Spaghetti: a round pasta that is the most commonly known pasta in America. It is available in thin and thick widths.

Tortellini: a small pasta that is stuffed and joined at the ends to form a ring; a larger version of capellitti.

Ziti: a short, tubular pasta similar to mostaccioli.

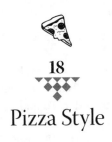

18

Pizza Style

Yes, pizza is Italian, but it has become Americanized, with toppings including barbecue chicken, ham, bacon, broccoli, spinach, and even cherries and Oreos. Pizza is available just about anywhere, including airports, food courts, sporting events, kid-focused activities, baseball games, and sit-down restaurants. Pizza is the number one choice for delivered food, for good reason: It's a favorite with every age group, it can be eaten hot or cold, and it's perfect for lunch, dinner, or late-night snacks (and some have been known to indulge in leftovers for breakfast). Pizza is so mainstream that it deserves its own chapter.

Many national chains, such as Pizza Hut, Godfather's Pizza, and Round Table Pizza, are focused on dine-in and take-out pizza. Some of the largest pizza purveyors, including Domino's, Papa John's, and Papa Murphy's Take 'n' Bake, offer pizza for take-out or delivery only. The Sbarro chain is found mostly in food courts and airports, and Chuck E. Cheese's caters to the younger set, merging playspace and pizza.

Then there are the more upscale, sit-down pizza establishments, which offer pizzas made in wood-fired or brick ovens and sport a wide array of unique toppings, such as goat's cheese, spinach, pesto, and roasted red peppers. Bertucci's, Uno's, and California Pizza Kitchen are three national chains, but plenty of independent pizzerias can be spotted on America's highways, byways, and city streets.

Pizza can be healthy—in fact healthier than a burger and fries—if you put the ten skills and strategies from Chapter 4 to work when placing your order. To make a healthy choice, keep in mind what you choose to top your pizza, the thickness of the crust, and—most importantly—how many pieces you eat. Overeating is the biggest problem with pizza. Put one or more of these portion-control strategies to work:

• Practice portion control from the start by ordering fewer slices or a smaller size.

• Stop eating when you're full and pack up the extra pieces to go.

Nutrition Snapshot

The following nutrition snapshot is intended to provide you with nutrition data for a variety of commonly pizza combos. All information shown below is for two pieces, which might be fewer slices than you usually eat. You'll see numbers that range from mind-blowing to healthy. Use them to educate yourself about the nutrition facts of your current pizza favorites. You may just find yourself changing your pizza orders and eating fewer slices.

Menu Item	Calories	Fat (g)	Saturated Fat (g)	*Trans* Fat (g)	Cholesterol (mg)	Sodium (mg)	Carbohydrate (g)	Protein (mg)
Classic with Mushrooms—12" (Domino's)	420	14	4	0	20	950	52	18
Classic with Extra Cheese—14" (Domino's)	640	21	5	0	40	1020	85	26

Menu Item	Calories	Fat (g)	Saturated Fat (g)	*Trans* Fat (g)	Cholesterol (mg)	Sodium (mg)	Carbohydrate (g)	Protein (mg)
Personal Pan Pepperoni—6" (Pizza Hut)	640	29	11	.5	22	1530	65	28
Thin Crust with Cheese—12" (Little Caesar's)	240	14	na	na	30	380	26	16
Veggie, Regular Crust—14" (Little Caesar's)	480	15	na	na	30	1420	64	24
Pepperoni, Regular Crust—16" (Little Caesar's)	480	17	na	na	40	900	54	24
Garden Special, Original Crust—12" (Papa John's)	560	18	5	0	30	1360	80	22
Garden Special, Thin Crust—12" (Papa John's)	400	14	4	0	20	890	56	16
All the Meats, Thin Crust—14" (Papa John's)	600	36	10	0	60	1400	46	26
Hand-Tossed Cheese—12" (Pizza Hut)	460	20	9	2	50	1240	50	24
Meat Lovers—12" (Pizza Hut)	740	44	8	0	90	1980	56	34
Stuffed Crust Supreme—14" (Pizza Hut)	780	38	16	3	100	2640	78	30
Hawaiian—14" (Donato's Pizza)	620	30	10	na	60	1780	58	30

The Pizza Profile

Think about it. What is pizza? The dough is basically flour, yeast, salt, and water, a combination that has no fat, no cholesterol, and few calories. Unfortunately, the large pizza chains have not yet introduced a whole-wheat crust, which could markedly increase the dietary fiber intake of Americans. (Whole-wheat crusts are available in the supermarket.) You may find an independent or small chain pizza establishment that offers the option of a whole grain crust. If it's available, order it. If not, ask for it. If the restaurant's management sees a significant demand for it, it may eventually appear on the menu. For example, a small New England chain called Geppetto's Grilled Pizzeria has introduced a crust with a higher level of high fiber-resistant starch called Hi-maize, which boosts the pizza's dietary fiber content and keeps white flour in the mix.

On top of the crust, tomato sauce is added, another low-calorie item. Some sauces may also contain some sugar and salt. Use your taste buds to determine the truth, compare nutrition information, read an ingredient list (large restaurant chains provide ingredient information on their web sites), or simply ask.

The next step is where the trouble begins: the cheese. Of course, it's high in calories and saturated and total fat.

The final step is adding toppings. Will they be low-calorie options like mushrooms, onions, spinach, and tomato slices, or high-fat choices, such as cheese, pepperoni, or sausage?

Thin, thick, stuffed crust, deep dish—the thickness of the crust is an essential decision. Most pizza restaurants offer a variety of choices. If calories are your biggest concern, thin crust is the way to go. Generally speaking, the thicker the crust, the higher the calorie count. Thicker crusts are also naturally higher in carbohydrates. If you prefer the thicker crust, eat fewer slices of pizza.

These days, particularly in upscale pizza restaurants, chefs are more creative with ingredient combinations used on pizza. That is great news for the nutrition-conscious, because some of these ingredients are vegetables and other lower-calorie foods (see the list under "Green Flag Toppings" on this page). The delicious taste of pizza can still be retained even if you reduce or remove the high-fat and less-than-healthy toppings of extra cheese, sausage, and pepperoni. Choose your toppings wisely: the more vegetables and lower-calorie items you choose, the healthier your pizza will be.

Before you order, think about how many pieces fit your needs—not wants. If you are trying to lose a few pounds, one or two slices are plenty. If cholesterol is your concern instead of calories, choose a vegetarian pizza, and three slices is about right. Order the right pizza size, so you have just enough for everyone's needs.

Another bit of advice: Enjoy a salad with your pizza. It takes care of at least one vegetable serving for the day and fills you up, leaving less room for pizza. Most sit-down restaurants that serve pizza also offer salads. Don't forget: The dressing should be served on the side. Chapter 13 provides all the information you need to keep your salads healthy.

▷ Green Flag Toppings

- △ green and red peppers
- △ roasted peppers
- △ onions
- △ sliced tomatoes
- △ mushrooms
- △ black olives
- △ broccoli
- △ eggplant

△ garlic

△ feta cheese

△ spinach

△ chicken

△ ham or Canadian bacon

△ anchovies

△ shrimp or crabmeat

△ artichoke hearts

▶ Red Flag Toppings

▼ extra cheese

▼ pepperoni

▼ sausage

▼ bacon

▼ meatballs

▼ prosciutto

▼ feta cheese

▼ Alfredo sauce

▼ mozzarella cheese

Special Requests

● "Please bring salad dressing on the side."

● "Can I have some vinegar on the side?"

● "Please go light on the cheese."

● "Can I substitute spicy chicken for the sausage (or pepperoni) on this pizza?"

● "Instead of the extra cheese, can you put on more onions and sliced tomatoes?"

● "Can I get this pizza without cheese?"

● "Please wrap this up so I can take it home."

● "Please bring a take-home box when you bring the pizza."

················· ◀ **"May I Take Your Order?"** ▶ ··················

Low-Calorie Sample Pizza Meal

Greek salad (green leaf lettuce with green pepper, tomato, and bits of feta cheese)
Quantity: 2 cups
Greek dressing
Quantity: 1 tbsp. (request lemon slices)
Pizza (topped with green peppers, broccoli, and onions)
Quantity: 1 slice from a large pizza

> **NUTRITION SUMMARY**
> 390 calories
> Carb: 49 g, 46%
> Fat: 15 g, 35%
> Protein: 19 g, 19%
> Cholesterol: 50 mg
> Sodium: 720 mg

Moderate-Calorie Sample Pizza Meal

Special-request salad (red leaf lettuce, green peppers, mushrooms, tomatoes, black olives, onion, and a sprinkle of mozzarella)
Quantity: 2 cups
Olive oil and vinegar dressing (on the side)
Quantity: 1 teaspoon oil; 2 tablespoons vinegar
Pizza (topped with sautéed chicken strips, roasted peppers, onions, white wine, oregano, feta cheese)
Quantity: 2 slices from large pizza

> **NUTRITION SUMMARY**
> 780 calories
> Carb: 81 g, 42%
> Fat: 31 g, 36%
> Protein: 43 g, 22%
> Cholesterol: 95 mg
> Sodium: 1170 mg

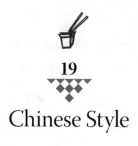

19

Chinese Style

Chinese foods, markets, and cooking styles were virtually unknown in America before the mid-1800s. Less than 200 years later, Chinese food is among the top three choices for ethnic food in America. When the Chinese first began to migrate to the United States, many settled in enclaves of major cities that become known as "Chinatowns." The streets of these neighborhoods were—and still are—dotted with many Chinese restaurants and bakeries.

In the past, Chinatowns were the only places to find Chinese food, but today it can be found just about everywhere: grocery stores, shopping malls, and urban, suburban, and even rural neighborhoods. Many Chinese restaurants are independently owned, but there is also a growing list of national chains, such as P.F. Chang's, Big Bowl, and Panda Express. LeeAnn Chin's, a Minneapolis-based chain, is a growing Asian-to-go option that touts the healthiness and *trans* fat-free qualities of its food. Many Chinese dishes, such as stir-fry chicken or vegetables and chop suey, also show up on family-fare restaurant menus.

Today, Chinese restaurants may specialize in one cuisine style—Szechuan, Hunan, Cantonese, or Peking, for example—or they may serve several or all of them. Many times, dishes on a Chinese menu will be named for the region from which they originate, such as Peking duck, Szechuan spicy chicken, and Hunan crispy beef.

Nutrition Snapshot

The following nutrition snapshot is intended to provide you with nutrition data for a handful of common menu items served at many Chinese restaurants. Just a few years ago, there was next to no nutrition information for Chinese restaurant foods because there were so few national chains. You'll see numbers that range from mind-blowing to healthy. Use this nutrition data, in addition to nutrition facts from Chinese foods you find on supermarket shelves, to make your best guess about what you are—and would be better off—eating at your favorite Chinese restaurants. You may just find yourself changing your orders.

Menu Item	Calories	Carbohy-drate (g)	Fat (g)	Saturated Fat (g)	*Trans* Fat (g)	Sodium (mg)
Hot and Sour Soup—1½ cup (Panda Express)	110	14	3.5	1	0	1370
A healthy choice. This fills you up and leaves less room for entrées.						
Chicken Egg Roll—1 (Panda Express)	170	17	8	2	0	410
Skip it. There are healthier appetizers, such as steamed dumplings (vegetable or pork), roast pork strips, or a bowl of soup.						
Beef with Broccoli—dinner portion (P.F. Changs)	1120	38	65	16	na	na
Pass on this and move on to a healthier choice.						
Orange Chicken—5.5 oz. (Panda Express)	500	42	27	6	1	810
Orange or orange peel in the name of the dish (whether it is poultry, beef, or shrimp) may sound healthy, but it should be a giveaway that the meat is fried before it's stir-fried, and that loads on the fat.						

Menu Item	Calories	Carbohydrate (g)	Fat (g)	Saturated Fat (g)	Trans Fat (g)	Sodium (mg)
Crispy Honey Shrimp—dinner portion (P.F. Changs)	1380	147	64	8	na	na
Do you have to wonder with a name like "crispy honey?" Yes, the calories and fat grams are more than enough for some people for an entire day. Skip it.						
Sweet and Sour Pork—dinner portion (P.F. Changs)	1100	106	46	14	na	na
Avoid sweet and sour dishes. The meat is breaded and fried, there are next to no vegetables, and the sauce is high in carbs.						
Mixed Vegetables—5.5 oz. (Panda Express)	70	6	4	1	0	170
A healthy choice. Enjoy it with white or brown rice or order it as a vegetable dish to complement a meat-focused dish.						
Lo Mein Combo—dinner portion (P.F. Changs)	1820	98	126	20	na	na
You might think the noodles would be healthy. Guess again. These noodles are tossed in a wok with oil and stir-fried with vegetables and meats. If lo mein is a must, get it with vegetables and split it several ways. Skip the rice if you enjoy lo mein.						
Fried Rice—8 oz. (Panda Express)	450	67	14	3	0	710
Stick to steamed white or brown rice.						

The Menu Profile

Many people think Chinese food is healthy because it is heavy on vegetables and light on fat. This perception may be true when these foods are prepared traditionally, but it's generally not true in Chinese restaurants in America. Both the way the foods are prepared and the ways in which they are eaten are different.

Chinese food in China is healthier than what's served in America. For example, protein (meats) are the focus for most Americans when they select dishes, whereas in China, the main focus is on carbohydrates, such as rice, noodles, and vegetables. Another reason is that Chinese food has been Americanized, which means added fat—fried noodles, fried appetizers, and battered and fried meats, such as shrimp and pork. Keep these points in mind when you order.

A Chinese meal can easily match the nutrition goals recommended for healthy eating—higher in carbohydrates and lower in protein, fat, and sodium. In addition, Chinese food has the potential to be low in saturated and *trans* fat and cholesterol. Rice and noodles are great sources of carbohydrates. Vegetables, which are also primarily carbohydrate, are abundant in Chinese cooking. You are familiar with many of the vegetables used: broccoli, cabbage, carrots, mushrooms, snowpeas, waterchestnuts, bamboo shoots, and onions. Others are less familiar, such as bok choy, napa cabbage, wood ears, and lily buds (see the section on Chinese Menu Lingo at the end of the chapter).

As with most foods, it is a challenge to limit the total amount of fat in the foods you order in Chinese restaurants, but it can be easier than in other types of restaurants, such as family-fare establishments. Special requests will help you limit the fatty foods, added oils, and high-sodium sauces, and special requests are easy because your food is usually made to order in both sit-down and take-out restaurants.

Avoid Chinese all-you-can-eat buffets and Chinese restaurants in food courts. You'll probably overeat, and you have no input on how dishes are prepared.

The most common Chinese cooking method is wok stir-frying. In fact, it used to be rare to find an oven in China. A wok can also be used for other cooking methods, such as braising and steaming. Wok cooking can be quite healthy. Minimal oil can be used, and foods are cooked only briefly so they retain their maximal vitamins and minerals.

Traditionally, much lard (pork fat) was used in Chinese cooking. Fortunately, healthier liquid oil is more commonplace today.

Peanut oil is the usual choice because of its high smoking point, which is an advantage when cooking at high temperatures in a wok. Peanut oil also gives dishes a slightly nutty flavor. It is primarily a monounsaturated fat, which is believed to help lower bad (LDL) cholesterol without lowering good (HDL) cholesterol. Sesame seed oil, which is a polyunsaturated fat, is also used, but in smaller quantities. Therefore, although Chinese cooking often uses plentiful oil, they are generally healthier choices.

One other villain is the high sodium content of Chinese food. Many dishes contain high-sodium soy sauces, light and dark, and monosodium glutamate (MSG). Other sauces, such as oyster, black bean, and hoisin, also contain large amounts of sodium. For a frame of reference, one tablespoon of soy sauce has about 1,000 milligrams of sodium, and the recommended daily intake is 2,300 milligrams!

A few special requests can quickly decrease the sodium. You can request that less soy and no MSG be used. Many Chinese restaurant menus boast that they do not use MSG. Chinese entrées are usually prepared when you order, so make your special requests. Do not try to eliminate soy sauce or sauces altogether, because the dish won't be as tasty. Consider using duck sauce, hot oil, chili sauce, or hot mustard as low-sodium flavorings that add some sweet taste or zip to your food. However, if you are watching your sodium intake closely, Chinese food might not be an optimal choice.

People with diabetes often find that Chinese food can wreak havoc with their blood glucose levels. That's not a surprise. There are lots of hidden carbohydrates in Chinese foods, from the sugar in marinades for meats to the corn starch that's used to thicken dishes before they are transferred from the wok to a serving platter. There are high-sugar sauces, including sweet-and-sour, hoisin, and duck. Ask the server to leave sugar and corn starch out of your dishes. (You may be told that it is already premixed into marinades or sauces.) Limit your intake of sugary sauces.

One of the biggest pluses of Chinese food is dishes are usually shared by everyone at the table. This is great for portion control. Don't feel compelled to order one dish per person. Instead, order fewer dishes than the number of people at the table. Order both meat- and vegetable-focused dishes. This balance can help you meet your healthy-eating goals.

In Chinese restaurants in America, you'll often be given fried Chinese noodles. Skip them. Many other Chinese appetizers are simply off-limits because they are fried: fried shrimp, wontons, chicken wings, and egg or spring rolls. Healthier appetizers are steamed Peking raviolis (choose vegetable or shrimp instead of pork), roast pork strips, and barbecued or teriyaki beef or chicken, if sodium is not a big concern.

Instead of the high-fat appetizers, fill up on a bowl of low-calorie broth-based soup (there are no creamy Chinese soups). Hot-and-sour, sizzling rice, or delights of three are all healthy soups, except for their sodium counts (hot-and-sour is usually the highest in sodium). Soup can help take the edge off your appetite, fill you up, and help you decrease the amount of food you eat for the rest of the meal.

Seafood is abundant on Chinese menus. Shrimp, prawns, scallops, calamari (squid), and whole or pieces of finfish are common. Other healthy protein foods are chicken and tofu (bean curd). Always be on the lookout for dishes with lots of vegetables. You might find the words "assorted vegetables" or "broccoli and water chestnuts." If it's not obvious, ask if a dish has vegetables, and if so, what kinds. Complement a meat dish with a vegetarian one. Good vegetarian dishes include spicy green beans, spinach and garlic, or vegetarian delight, but skip

Szechuan eggplant—it's loaded with fat. Always make sure none of the ingredients in the dish are deep-fried.

On to the rice and noodles: Both are always available, and some healthy and some are not. Steamed brown rice is ideal and is becoming available in more Chinese restaurants, but it is still unavailable in many places. Steamed white rice with no added salt or fats is more common. Fried rice is white rice stir-fried (which adds oil) with soy sauce (which adds sodium) that turns it brown. If you order fried rice, stick with the vegetable variety and avoid the fat and protein added by pork or other meats. Similar advice holds true for lo mein and pan-fried noodles—order a vegetable selection instead of one with meat. The basic noodle is healthy, but the health quotient goes downhill as chefs add oils and high-sodium sauces. Eat only a small amount of these dishes.

Desserts are often afterthoughts in Chinese restaurants, but pineapple and orange sections or lychee nuts with fortune cookies may appear on your table. A dessert menu might include ice cream or fried bananas; both should be skipped. You'd also be wise to read your fortune and leave the cookie.

Chopsticks are the eating utensils of choice, but forks and spoons are also available. However, a lack of aptitude with chopsticks might be a blessing in disguise: Your lack of dexterity will slow your pace of eating.

▷ Green Flag Words

The asterisks (*) denote foods that are high in sodium.

Ingredients

△ bean curd (tofu) (get it sautéed, but not fried)
△ assorted vegetables, such as broccoli, mushrooms, onions, carrots, cabbage, water chestnuts, bamboo shoots, lily buds, wood ears, and bean sprouts

△ fish, shrimp, scallops, squid
△ chicken, roast pork
△ pineapple
△ tomatoes
△ soy sauce,* hoisin sauce, plum sauce*
△ Chinese hot mustard
△ hot oil
△ chili sauce
△ sweet (duck) sauce
△ broth (for both-based soups)
△ Chinese spices
△ ginger
△ garlic

Cooking Methods/Menu Descriptions/Names

△ brown sauce*
△ oyster sauce, black bean sauce*
△ light wine sauce
△ lobster sauce
△ simmered or braised
△ steamed
△ stir-fried with vegetables
△ hot and spicy tomato sauce
△ served on sizzling platter
△ slippery white sauce or velvet sauce
△ moo shi (or moo shu)
△ chow mein
△ chop suey

▶ Red Flag Words

Ingredients

- ▼ duck
- ▼ cashews or peanuts
- ▼ pieces of egg
- ▼ water chestnut flour
- ▼ bits of pork or egg
- ▼ Chinese noodles

Cooking Methods/Menu Descriptions/Names

- ▼ fried or deep-fried
- ▼ battered or breaded and fried
- ▼ deep-fried until crispy
- ▼ crispy
- ▼ served in bird's nest
- ▼ sweet-and-sour
- ▼ spare ribs
- ▼ orange peel, orange, or lemon chicken or beef (usually deep fried)
- ▼ whole fish (usually fried)
- ▼ Kung Pao

At the Table

- ▼ Chinese noodles

Special Requests

- ◆ "Please remove the crispy fried noodles from the table."
- ◆ "Please don't use MSG."
- ◆ "What type of oil is used for stir-frying?" (If lard or other saturated fat, request that peanut or another non-animal fat be used.)

♦ "Would it be possible to use less oil in the preparation?"
♦ "Can you sauté the chicken (or other meat) instead of breading and deep-frying it?"
♦ "Would it be possible to use less soy sauce?"
♦ "Can you substitute chicken in this dish for the duck?"
♦ "Could you substitute (or add more) broccoli?"
♦ "Please don't garnish my meal with peanuts or cashews."
♦ "Can you leave out the crispy fried wontons?"
♦ "Can you leave out the cornstarch?"

Typical Menu: Chinese Style

✿ *Indicates preferred choices*
✦ *Indicates hot and spicy dish*

Appetizers

Egg rolls
Spring rolls
✿ **Steamed Peking raviolis**
✿ **Peking raviolis (vegetable)**
✿ **Roast pork strips**
Barbecued spareribs
✿ **Teriyaki,** beef or chicken on skewers
Jumbo shrimp, fried
Wontons, fried

Soups

✿ **Hot-and-sour**
✿ **Wonton**
✿ **Sizzling rice and chicken or shrimp**
✿ **Delights of three** (assorted Chinese vegetables and chicken, pork, and beef strips)
✿ **Egg drop**

✿ **Chicken and corn soup** (chicken broth with egg, chicken and corn)

Poultry

✿ **Velvet chicken** (breast of chicken, snow peas, water chestnuts, bamboo shoots, and garnish of egg white)

✚ **General Tsao's chicken** (cubes of chicken coated with water chestnut flour and eggs, deep-fried until crispy, and coated with hot ginger sauce). (Note: Getting the chicken sautéed helps decrease the fat, but the hot ginger sauce is still high in calories.)

Sweet-and-sour chicken (battered and fried chicken topped with a thick, sweet, and pungent sauce and pineapple)

✿ **Chicken chop suey** (breast of chicken stir-fried with celery, Chinese cabbage, and assorted vegetables)

✿ **Sizzling sliced chicken with vegetables** (sliced breast of chicken with assorted Chinese vegetables)

✚ **Yu Hsiang chicken** (strips of chicken stir-fried with bamboo shoots, water chestnuts, wood ears, lily buds, and Chinese cabbage)

Sweet-and-pungent duck (cubes of battered, deep-fried duck served with water chestnuts, cherries, and peas)

Orange chicken (deep-fried pieces of chicken tossed with chili peppers and fresh orange peel)

Seafood

✿ **Shrimp** with broccoli and mushrooms (stir-fried shrimp with broccoli and Chinese mushrooms in a light egg-white sauce)

✚ **Spicy crispy whole fish** (a whole fish deep-fried and coated with a hot, spicy sauce)

Shrimp and cashews (whole shrimp stir-fried with cashew nuts and water chestnuts)

✦ **Szechuan-style fresh fish fillets** (deep fried fish fillets sautéed with bamboo shoots and scallions and served with a hot and spicy sauce)

✿ **Moo shu shrimp** (stir-fried shrimp with Chinese vegetables, served with Chinese pancakes and hoisin sauce)

Meats

✿ **Beef and broccoli** with black mushrooms (strips of beef sautéed with broccoli and black mushrooms in oyster sauce)

✦ **Orange beef** (deep-fried beef tossed with chili peppers and fresh orange peel)

✿ **Twice-cooked pork** (pork with cabbage, green peppers, and bamboo shoots in a hot bean sauce)

✦ **Hunan crispy beef** (deep-fried beef coated with a hot Hunan sauce and served with broccoli)

✿ **Roast pork** with vegetables (slices of stir-fried pork with assorted Chinese vegetables)

✿ **Beef chow mein** (sliced stir-fried beef with diced cabbage, onions, sliced mushrooms, and other Chinese vegetables)

Kung Pao beef (stir-fried beef in a dark sauce with chili peppers, peanuts, and Chinese vegetables)

Vegetables

✿ **Vegetarian delight** (crunchy stir-fried vegetables in a light sauce)

✦ **Yu Hsiang eggplant** (stir-fried eggplant with other Chinese vegetables)

✿ **Spicy green beans** (green beans sautéed in hot and spicy Hunan sauce)

✿ **Broccoli and black mushrooms** (in oyster sauce)
✿ **Spinach and garlic** (stir-fried spinach with garlic)

Rice

✿ **Steamed white or brown rice**
Pork- or beef-fried rice
Vegetable-fried rice

Noodles

Roast pork lo mein
Chicken lo mein
Vegetable lo mein
Pan-fried noodles (with shrimp, pork, and chicken)
Pan-fried noodles (with assorted Chinese vegetables)

Desserts

✿ **Pineapple chunks**
✿ **Lychee nuts**
Vanilla ice cream
Fried bananas (served with sweet syrup sauce)
✿ **Fortune cookies**

⟨ "May I Take Your Order?" ⟩

Low-Calorie Sample Meal

Hot-and-sour soup
Quantity: 1 cup
Exchanges: 1 vegetable
Yu Hsiang chicken
Quantity: 1 cup (½ order)
Shrimp with broccoli and mushrooms
Quantity: 1 cup (½ order)
Steamed white rice
Quantity: ⅔ cup
Fortune cookie
Read your fortune and skip the cookie.

> **NUTRITION SUMMARY**
> 570 calories
> Carb: 51 g, 36%
> Fat: 22 g, 35%
> Protein: 41 g, 29%
> Cholesterol: 150 mg
> Sodium: 1300 mg

Moderate-Calorie Sample Meal

Peking raviolis, vegetable, steamed
Quantity: 2
Moo-shu shrimp
Quantity: 2 pancakes and ½ cup of filling in each pancake (½ order)
Vegetable lo mein noodles
Quantity: 1 cup (½ order)
Tsingtao beer
Quantity: 12 oz.

> **NUTRITION SUMMARY**
> 920 calories
> Carb: 113 g, 49%
> Fat: 25 g, 24%
> Protein: 44 g, 19%
> Alcohol: 8% calories
> Cholesterol: 134 mg
> Sodium: 1300 mg

Chinese Menu Lingo

Bean curd: known as "tofu" to Americans, it is made of soybeans and formed into cubes. It is used in soups and many other dishes. Be careful to request that it not be fried.

Black bean sauce: a thick, brown sauce made of fermented soybeans, salt, and wheat flour that is frequently used in Cantonese cooking.

Bok choy: also known as Chinese chard, it looks like a cross between celery and cabbage.

Five-spice powder: a reddish-brown powder that combines star anise, fennel, cinnamon, cloves, and Szechuan pepper. Used in Szechuan dishes.

Hoisin sauce: a sweet-and-spicy thick sauce made from soybeans, sugar, garlic, chili, and vinegar and served with moo shu dishes. Also called plum sauce.

Lily buds: dried, golden-colored buds with a light, flowery flavor that are used in entrées and soups. Also called lotus or tiger lily buds.

Lychees or lychee nuts: a crimson-colored fruit with translucent flesh around a brown seed.

Monosodium glutamate (MSG): a white powder used in small amounts to bring out and enhance the flavors of ingredients.

Napa: also referred to as Chinese cabbage, it has thick-ribbed stalks and crinkled leaves.

Oyster sauce: a rich, thick sauce made of oysters, their cooking liquid, and soy sauce that is frequently used in Cantonese dishes.

Plum sauce: a thick amber-colored sauce made from plums, apricots, hot peppers, vinegar, and sugar, it has a spicy sweet-and-sour flavor.

Sesame seed oil: oil extracted from sesame seeds. It has a strong sesame flavor and is used as seasoning for soups, seafood, and other dishes.

Soy sauce: either light or dark, it is used in lieu of salt in virtually all Chinese dishes.

Sweet-and-sour sauce: a thick sauce made from sugar, vinegar, and soy sauce. Meat, chicken, or shrimp served in this sauce has usually been dipped in batter and fried.

Wood ear: a variety of tree lichen that is brown and resembles a wrinkled ear that is used in some soups and vegetable dishes. It is soaked before use.

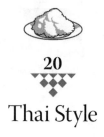

20

Thai Style

Only 20 years ago, Thai restaurants were a rarity in the U.S. Today, restaurants serving Thai food or Asian fusion cuisine with a sampling of Thai specialties are common nationwide. So far, there are no Thai chain restaurants; most are independently run with just one or a few locations.

Americans have become more familiar with such Thai dishes as tod mun, shrimp choo chee, and a favorite noodle dish on nearly every Thai menu—pad Thai. Thai food can be reasonably healthy—light on fats, meats, and sauces, and moderate on healthy carbs such as vegetables, noodles, and rice. Like other Asian cuisines, it's easier to share and use other strategies to avoid overeating.

Thai cuisine is often compared with Chinese, but the primary similarities are stir-frying, the central role of rice, and a cadre of similar meat and vegetable ingredients. Thai food differs from Chinese food substantially because of the many different herbs and spices, and the fact that most Thai dishes are based with fish sauce rather than soy sauce. In terms of taste, Thai food more closely resembles Indian fare, with its many curries and its use of aromatic flavors and spices like coriander, cumin, cardamom, and cinnamon, to name a few.

Nutrition Snapshot

The following nutrition snapshot is intended to provide you with the nutrition numbers for a handful of common menu items served at Thai restaurants. Unfortunately, little nutrition data is available for Thai restaurant food because most Thai restaurants are independently owned. For the sampling of Thai offerings listed below, you'll see nutrition numbers that range from mind-blowing to healthy. Use this data to educate yourself about the nutrition makeup of your current favorites in Thai restaurants. If necessary, consider changing your orders to eat healthier.

Menu Item	Calories	Carbohy-drate (g)	Fat (g)	Saturated Fat (g)	*Trans* Fat (g)	Sodium (mg)
Tom Yam (Hot & Sour) Soup with Seafood—1 cup (www.calorie king.com)	100	4	3	na	na	na
A healthy and filling choice.						
Fried Rice—1 serving (Hibachi-San Japanese Grill)	470	77	14	3	na	600
This version is lowfat and has a reasonable amount of sodium. It won't always be so.						
Brown Rice—1 serving (Chin's Asia Fresh)	68	15	.5	na	na	na
A healthy choice. When brown rice is available, request it.						
Thai Peanut Lo Mein, Pork—1 serving (Chin's Asia Fresh)	164	18	8	na	na	na
This is a small but healthy serving.						
Thai Chicken Curry with Ginger—1 cup (www.calorie king.com)	390	4	34	na	na	na
High in fat, probably because of the coconut milk.						
Thai Spring Roll—1 (www.calorie king.com)	110	13	6	na	na	na
The small serving makes this an acceptable choice.						

Menu Item	Calories	Carbohydrate (g)	Fat (g)	Saturated Fat (g)	*Trans* Fat (g)	Sodium (mg)
Thai Beef Salad without Dressing—1 serving (www.calorie king.com)	260	15	9	na	na	na
A healthy choice.						
Thai Peanut with Tofu—1 dish (Chin's Asia Fresh)	264	14	18	na	na	na
A healthy choice.						
Indo Coconut Curry with Pork—1 serving (Chin's Asia Fresh)	170	11	9	na	na	na
A healthy choice.						
Pad Thai with Beef—1 serving (Chin's Asia Fresh)	403	49	12.5	na	na	na
A healthy choice.						

The Menu Profile

Although Thai cooking is generally light and healthy, fat does creep in from various sources. Fried entrées are fairly uncommon, but many of the appetizers, are deep-fried. Most often, entrées are stir-fried in a liquid oil. If you frequent a particular Thai restaurant, ask what type of oil it uses.

Coconut milk is used in most Thai curry dishes. Unfortunately, coconut milk, like coconut oil, contains saturated fat and a hefty dose of calories. A quarter-cup of coconut milk—the amount you might have in a half-portion of a Thai curry dish—contains 120 calories (most of which is calories from fat), 13 grams of fat and 11 grams of saturated fat. For this reason, it is generally wise to avoid curry entrées and soups that are not clear.

Like Chinese food, Thai food can be high in sodium. The spicing and flavoring is not as dependent on soy sauce as Chinese cuisine, but it is not uncommon to see soy sauce and/or salt added to main dishes, soups, rice (other than steamed), and noodle dishes. Some sauces, such as yellow bean paste, shrimp paste, and fish sauce (which is an ingredient in most Thai dishes), also add sodium.

People with diabetes should be advised that sugar is used in many dishes. On average, one teaspoon to two tablespoons of sugar are added to most dishes. If you notice that your blood glucose generally rises after eating Thai food, adjust your medication if you are able, limit certain items that add sugars and starches, and use the portion control technique to eat fewer high-sugar and high-carbohydrate foods.

Thai dishes in sit-down restaurants are generally made to order. This makes special requests easier to grant—so make them. Some suggestions: "Don't fry the tofu before putting it in the dish," or "Please sauté the shrimp rather than deep-frying it before you put it in the dish." Family-style eating is common-place, which allows you to share items and control portions.

For healthy appetizers, try beef or chicken satay, nonfried basil or vegetable rolls, or steamed seafood. But beware the tasty sauces. Peanut sauce, which is served with satay, is loaded with fat. Request a lighter sauce, such as a tamarind sweet-and-sour sauce, with basil or vegetable rolls. Thai rolls, tod mun, and stuffed chicken wings are deep-fried, but the portions are small. If you've got a few calories to spare and dining companions to share with, indulge in a few tastes. If not, just dive into the soups and entrées.

Thai soups are delicious and filling, and they take the edge off your appetite. Clear-broth soups, like tom yum koong and pok taek, have a bit of protein and great taste from Thai spices such as lemon grass, chili paste, and lime juice. Their calorie count is low, but the sodium is high. Avoid tom ka gai, or chicken coconut, because it contains coconut milk. Stick with soups you can see through.

Salads are unusual for some Southeast Asian cuisines but are regularly found on Thai menus. Thai salads range from simple garden salads to salads that combine unusual ingredients, such as green papaya and dried shrimp. Other salads combine vegetables and/or fruit with beef, chicken, or seafood.

Salad dressings are light and made with flavorings like lemon grass, chilies, lime juice, and sometimes peanut sauce. Remember to ask for dressing on the side. You may wish to request tamarind, a light sweet-and-sour dressing. If your dining companions are eating fried appetizers, a salad is a smart choice. Another option is to order a seafood or beef salad with a bowl of steamed rice as your main course. You can share it with your dining companions as one of the group's entrée choices.

You'll find many healthy entrées in any Thai restaurant. Complement a protein-dense dish with one packed with veggies. Find a vegetable and tofu (bean curd) dish to help you moderate your animal protein and saturated fat. (Remember to make sure the tofu is not fried.)

It's common to see peanuts, cashews, or peanut sauce as additions to Thai dishes. If you are concerned about fat content, tell the server to leave them in the kitchen. If you want a few grams of healthier fats, leave them on. If calories are a prime concern, basil, chili, lime juice, and curry-paste sauces are lower in calories.

Curry dishes often contain coconut milk, which adds lots of saturated fat. The best advice is to share or skip curry sauces—yellow, green, red, or mussaman. Order one curry dish to share with a group. Minimize the amount of sauce you spoon on. Ask that your curry be packed with extra veggies, such as broccoli, green beans, and carrots.

Most menus offer many rice and noodle dishes. The smartest choice is steamed white rice. It's long grain, often with a sprinkling of jasmine grains. Fried rice, which is a bit lighter in both fat and color than Chinese fried rice, is also available. Thai fried rice comes in varieties such as vegetable, beef, chicken, pork, seafood, or a combination of several. If you must have fried rice, stick with vegetable, and only eat a small amount.

Pad Thai is stir-fried noodles with finely chopped peanuts, bean sprouts, egg, tofu, scallions and often a slice of lime on the side. Vegetarian pad Thai comes with tofu; you can also choose chicken or shrimp varieties. Like fried rice, it is made with oil, and thus it has a fair amount of fat and calories. Enjoy it along with steamed rice, or only eat a small portion and share the rest with dining companions. Other noodle dishes, such as drunken noodles, spend time in a wok being tossed with oil and sodium-laden sauces, so use the same strategies suggested for pad Thai.

The dessert listings in most Thai restaurants are easy to pass up. You might find lychee, a common Southeast Asian fruit, and puddings or custards. Lychee is fine, but a relaxing cup of coffee or tea might satisfy you just as much—with fewer calories.

Most Thai restaurants offer Thai ice coffee or ice tea. Don't be fooled into thinking these are just coffee or tea—they also contain plenty of sugar and milk or cream. If one will satisfy your sweet tooth and you've got the calories to spend, it's not a terrible choice, but if you can resist, you should.

▷ Green Flag Words

Ingredients

△ basil or basil leaves

△ lemon grass

△ mint or mint leaves

△ lime juice, kafir limes

△ green papaya

△ pineapple

△ chili, chili paste, crushed dried chili

△ Thai spices

△ fish sauce

△ sweet-and-sour sauce

△ bean-thread noodles

△ napa (cabbage), bamboo shoots, black mushrooms (other vegetables)

△ green beans, broccoli, carrots, tomatoes

△ scallops, shrimp, squid, chicken

△ bed of spinach or mixed vegetables

Cooking Methods/Menu Descriptions/Names

△ stir-fried

△ sautéed

△ sizzling

△ braised

△ marinated

△ barbecued

△ clear broth soup

△ basil sauce

△ lime sauce

△ Thai salad

▶ Red Flag Words

Ingredients

▼ topped with peanuts, ground peanuts

▼ topped with cashews

▼ coconut milk

- ▼ fried tofu
- ▼ roasted duck (skin and fat usually left on)

Cooking Methods/Menu Descriptions/Names

- ▼ golden brown
- ▼ fried
- ▼ deep-fried
- ▼ crispy
- ▼ coconut milk soup
- ▼ mee-krob (crispy noodles)
- ▼ red, green, yellow, or mussaman curry sauce
- ▼ served with peanut sauce

Special Requests

- ◗ "Please put the dressing on the side of the salad."
- ◗ "Please bring extra plates. We are going to share all the items."
- ◗ "Please hold the peanuts (or cashews) on this dish."
- ◗ "Can I get tamarind sauce (or other light appetizer dipping sauce) instead of peanut sauce with the appetizer?"
- ◗ "What oil is used to prepare your foods?" (If it's coconut oil or lard, ask that vegetable oil be used instead.)
- ◗ "Please minimize the salt and soy (or fish) sauce. I'm carefully watching my sodium consumption."
- ◗ "Can I substitute scallops for shrimp or beef in this dish?"
- ◗ "Could I have more vegetables in this dish?"
- ◗ "Can you please sauté the tofu instead of deep-frying it?"
- ◗ "Could I get the rest of this wrapped up to take home? I'd like to enjoy it for dinner tomorrow night."
- ◗ "Please make this dish hot. I like lots of flavor."

Typical Menu: Thai Style

✿ *Indicates preferred choices*

Appetizers

Thai spring rolls (vegetable-filled, deep-fried, and served with sweet-and-sour sauce)

✿ **Basil vegetable rolls** (garden fresh vegetables rolled with basil leaves and served with sweet-and-sour sauce)

✿ **Basil shrimp rolls** (garden fresh vegetables rolled with shrimp and basil leaves and served with sweet-and-sour sauce)

✿ **Satay** (beef or chicken marinated in coconut milk and curry, barbecued on skewers, and served with peanut sauce and cucumber salad) (Note: Use the peanut sauce sparingly, and chicken satay is a better choice than beef.)

Tod mun (minced shrimp and codfish mixed with Thai curry, fried until golden brown, and served with cucumber sauce)

✿ **Steamed mussels** (steamed with lemon grass, sweet basil leaves, chili, and Thai spices and served with chili sauce)

✿ **Seafood kebab** (shrimp, scallops, and vegetables served with hot sauce on skewers)

Mee-krob (sweet crispy rice noodles with shrimp, chicken, and bean sprouts)

Soups

✿ **Tom yum koong** (Thai shrimp soup with lemon grass, chili paste, lime juice, and straw mushrooms)

Tom ka gai (chicken in coconut milk soup with mushrooms and lime juice)

✿ **Crystal noodles** (clear soup with chicken, bean-thread noodles, and vegetables)

Salads

- ✵ **Thai salad** (green mixed garden salad with tofu and egg wedges, dressed with a spiced peanut sauce)
- ✵ **Papaya salad** (fresh green papaya with garlic, tomato, green beans, Thai chili, and ground peanuts tossed in spicy lime juice with dried shrimp)
- ✵ **Pla koong** (spicy shrimp salad with onions, scallions, tomatoes, mushrooms, and lemon grass, all tossed with chili and lime juice)
- ✵ **Spiced beef salad** (charbroiled beef slices in a chili paste with lemon grass, lettuce, tomatoes, mushrooms, and scallions, tossed in a spicy lemon dressing)
- ✵ **Yam yai** (a spicy combination salad of shrimp, pork, and chicken with lettuce, cucumber, onions, and tomato in a light, spicy dressing)

Curry

The following curry dishes can be made with chicken, beef, shrimp, scallops, tofu, or vegetables. If you order tofu, ask that it not be deep fried.

- * **Green curry** (in coconut milk, with bamboo shoots, green peppers, string beans, green peas, and zucchini)
- * **Red curry** (in coconut milk, with bamboo shoots and red and green peppers)
- * **Mussaman curry** (in coconut milk, with potatoes, onions, carrots, and peanuts) (Note: This is the heaviest of the curries and is often served with beef. The others contain more vegetables and are lighter.)

* Note comments in text about coconut milk.

Poultry

Crispy duck (roasted duck, steamed with soy sauce, topped with fried spinach, and served with plum sauce)

Chili duck (sautéed roast duck with onion, hot peppers, mushrooms, scallions, fresh sweet basil leaves, and spiced tomato sauce)

✿ **Thai chicken** (chicken sautéed with cashews, onions, mushrooms, pineapple, tomatoes, scallions, and chili)

✿ **Pad pak** (sautéed sliced chicken on a bed of broccoli, carrots, cauliflower, green beans, and asparagus; also available with shrimp)

✿ **Pad prik king** (sautéed chicken with chili paste, green beans, Kafir lime, and basil; also available with beef or pork)

Beef/Pork

* **Spareribs curry** (a red coconut curry with boneless spareribs, peas, string beans, snow peas, hot pepper, tomato, and sweet basil leaves)

✿ **Beef basil** (sautéed beef, flavored with hot basil leaves, fresh hot peppers, mushrooms, and red peppers)

Praram long song (fried beef with a special curry sauce and peanuts over a bed of spinach)

✿ **Ginger pork** (sautéed pork in ginger with green peppers, onions, scallions, mushrooms, and chili paste)

* Note comments in text about coconut milk.

Seafood

Hot Thai fish (a deep-fried catfish fillet topped with bamboo shoots, baby corn, mushrooms, eggplant, hot chili, basil leaves, and Thai spices)

✲ **Garlic shrimp** (shrimp sautéed with fresh garlic, peppercorns, snow peas, and napa and served on a bed of sliced cucumbers)
✲ **Poy sian** (seafood sautéed with straw mushrooms, napa, bamboo shoots, onions, and string beans)
✲ **Scallops bamboo** (sea scallops sautéed with bamboo shoots, snow peas, baby corn, mushrooms, scallions, and Thai spices)
Soft shell crabs (deep-fried soft-shell crab topped with chili, onion, and basil)

Vegetables

Royal tofu (deep-fried pieces of tofu with snow peas, onions, scallions, broccoli, and a spicy chili sauce)
✲ **Red curry vegetables** (broccoli, cabbage, carrots, and green beans topped with a spicy red curry sauce)
✲ **Pad jay** (napa, celery, onions, carrots, mushrooms, and bean sprouts topped with a sauce of Thai spices)

Rice and Noodles

Fried rice (white rice stir-fried with chicken, scallions, green peas, onions, and egg)
Vegetable fried rice (white rice stir-fried with assorted stir-fry vegetables)
✲ **Steamed rice**
Pad Thai (noodles stir-fried with ground peanuts, bean sprouts, egg, tofu, and scallions; sometimes includes chicken or shrimp)
Drunken noodles (stir-fried wide rice noodles, ground chili, peppers, onions, bean spouts, Chinese broccoli, and basil)

Desserts

✤ **Lychee nuts**

Fried bananas (deep-fried bananas served with a sweet
syrup sauce)

Thai custard

················ ◀ **"May I Take Your Order?"** ▶ ················

Low-Calorie Sample Meal

Tom yun koong
Quantity: 1 cup
Thai chicken (hold cashews)
Quantity: 1 cup (½ order)
Poy sian
Quantity: 1 cup (½ order)
Steamed rice
Quantity: ⅔ cup
Mineral water
Quantity: 12 oz.
Exchanges: free

NUTRITION SUMMARY
550 calories
Carb: 67 g, 49%
Fat: 18 g, 29%
Protein: 30 g, 22%
Cholesterol: 153 mg
Sodium: 1210 mg

Moderate-Calorie Sample Meal

Green curry with tofu
Quantity: 1 cup (½ order)
Scallops bamboo
Quantity: 1 cup (½ order)
Pad Thai
Quantity: 1 cup
Steamed rice
Quantity: ⅔ cup
Coffee
Quantity: 1 cup

NUTRITION SUMMARY
820 calories
Carb: 86 g, 42%
Fat: 32 g, 35%
Protein: 47 g, 23%
Cholesterol: 64 mg
Sodium: 1260 mg

Thai Menu Lingo

Bamboo shoots: an Asian vegetable commonly found in Thai entrées that is light in color, crunchy, stringy in texture, and very low in calories.

Basil: called horapa in Thailand, it is mainly used in leaf form in Thai dishes; there are several types of basil used in Thai recipes.

Cardamom: a member of the ginger family, its whole or ground seeds are often used in curry mixtures and other dishes.

Chilies: there are various types with varying degrees of hotness. Red and green are common and are used whole, chopped, or ground into paste for sauces. Chilies add zip with almost no calories. Chili icons on Thai menus often denote the level of hotness of dishes or how much chili is used.

Cilantro: a member of the carrot family, it is also called Chinese parsley or coriander (it is actually the leaves of the coriander plant). Cilantro is widely used in Mexican, Caribbean, and Asian cooking. Cilantro looks like Italian parsley, but its leaves are more delicate.

Coconut milk: a liquid extracted when fresh coconut is grated. It is not the liquid from inside the coconut. Coconut milk is used for marinating (such as with satay) and in sauces for various dishes, such as curry sauces. It is high in saturated fat and calories.

Coriander: dried coriander seed is a primary ingredient in curry mixtures. The seeds or leaves (cilantro) of the plant are also used as an essential spice in Thai recipes.

Cumin: a fragrant spice important to curry mixtures, used either as seeds or ground.

Curry: a combination of spices; different spice and food combinations create the green, red, and mussaman curry mixtures.

Kapi: a dried shrimp paste made from prawns or shrimp that is commonly used to flavor Thai dishes.

Lemon grass: takrai, as it's known in Thailand, is an Asian plant whose bulbous base is used to add a lemony flavor to many soups and main entrées. It is cut into strips and is fibrous in nature.

Lime: called makrut in Thai, lime leaves or the juices of kafir limes are commonly used in soups, salads, and entrées.

Nam pla: a fish sauce. It is Thai food's answer to soy sauce; this thin, high-sodium brown sauce brings out the flavor of other foods.

Nam prik: called Thai shrimp sauce, it is used to flavor many Thai foods. It is made of shrimp paste, chilies, lime juice, soy sauce, and sugar.

Napa: also referred to as Chinese cabbage, it has thickribbed stalks and crinkled leaves.

Palm sugar: a strong-flavored, dark sugar obtained from the sap of coconut palms. It is boiled down until it crystallizes.

Scallions: also called spring onions, they are white, slender, and have long green stems. They are usually chopped into short or long pieces and stir-fried into dishes.

Soy sauce: a sauce made from soybeans that adds a salty flavor to many Thai dishes.

Tamarind: an acidic fruit known for its tart flavor.

Turmeric: the spice that lends the yellow-orange color to commercial curry, it is a member of the ginger family.

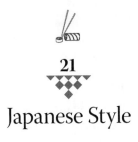

21

Japanese Style

Years ago, Japanese restaurants were hard to find, but today, Japanese restaurants can be found all over in America, in metropolitan areas, suburbs, airports, and food courts. The menu offerings—both in type and quantity—vary. Many traditional Japanese restaurants serve a range of Japanese favorites, such as tempura, sukiyaki, and teriyaki, and lesser-known dishes, such as agemono, yosenabe, and donburi. These restaurants may also feature a busy sushi bar, with several sushi chefs rolling up familiar and exotic rolls. In fact, many Japanese restaurants only serve sushi. As sushi is a generally healthy and portable food, sushi chain restaurants like Bumblefish (which bills itself as "neo-Asian fast food") are opening up.

Another category of Japanese restaurants that are particularly popular with kids—and therefore families—are Japanese steak houses, such as Benihana. In these restaurants, the spotlight is on acrobatic chefs who prepare tempting chicken, shrimp, or beef dishes table-side. It is now commonplace to find Japanese preparations on family-fare restaurant menus and the menus of upscale restaurants serving a fusion of cuisines.

For the most part, Japanese food is both healthy and lowfat. It is focused on vegetables, moderate on starches, and light on seafood, meats, dairy products, and fats. The biggest thorn in the side of Japanese cuisine is its high sodium count and a few deep-fried items, the best known of which is tempura.

Nutrition Snapshot

The following nutrition snapshot provides two charts for Japanese food. The first provides the nutrition numbers for a handful of common sushi offerings. The second chart provides the nutrition numbers for some common items served at Japanese restaurants. There continues to be a minimal amount of nutrition information for Japanese restaurant foods. One reason is that most Japanese restaurants, other than the few Japanese steak house chains, are independent restaurants. However, as more chain Japanese sushi bars or full scale restaurants blossom, the availability of nutrition information should increase as well. Generally speaking the nutrition numbers for Japanese food are reasonably healthy, that is other than the sodium counts or the fat count on a few items which are easy to steer clear from. Put these to use to educate yourself about the nutrition makeup of your current order in these restaurants and, if need be, begin to make changes to eat healthier.

Sushi

Menu Item	Calories	Carbohydrate (g)	Fat (g)	Saturated Fat (g)	*Trans* Fat (g)	Sodium (mg)
Cucumber Roll—1 serving/8 pieces (Bumblefish)	264	57	0	0	na	142
A healthy choice.						
Cucumber Roll—8 pcs. (www.sushifaq.com)	136	30	0	0	na	na
A healthy choice.						

Menu Item	Calories	Carbohy-drate (g)	Fat (g)	Saturated Fat (g)	*Trans* Fat (g)	Sodium (mg)
Crab and Shrimp Roll—1 serving / 8 pcs. (Bumblefish)	230	45	3	0	na	449
A healthy choice.						
Eel Roll—1 serving /8 pcs. (Bumblefish)	281	37	9	2	na	422
A healthy choice, and you get some omega-3 fats.						
California Roll—8 pcs. (Hibachi-San Japanese Grill)	450	75	11	2	na	1580
A healthy choice, but a bit higher in fat and high in sodium.						
Assorted Sushi—6 pcs. (Hibachi-San Japanese Grill)	290	51	2	0	na	820
A healthy choice.						
Shrimp Tempura Roll—6 pcs. (www.sushifaq.com)	508	64	21	na	na	na
The fat count goes up because the shrimp is fried.						
Spicy Tuna Roll—10 pcs (Hibachi-San Japanese Grill)	450	67	7	2	na	1230
A healthy choice.						
Eel and Avocado Roll—8 pcs. (www.sushifaq.com)	372	31	17	na	na	na
The fat is high because of the eel and avocado. Although they are higher in fat, the ingredients are healthy.						
Tuna Roll—8 pcs. (www.sushifaq.com)	184	27	2	na	na	na
A healthy choice.						

Nonsushi Menu Items

Menu Item	Calories	Carbohy-drate (g)	Fat (g)	Saturated Fat (g)	*Trans* Fat (g)	Sodium (mg)
Fried Rice—1 serving (Hibachi-San Japanese Grill)	470	77	14	3	na	600
A healthy choice.						
Teriyaki Udon, Beef—1 bowl (2½ servings) (Chin's Asia Fresh)	427	51	12	na	na	na
A healthy choice, but probably high in sodium.						
Teriyaki Udon, Beef—1 serving (Chin's Asia Fresh)	170	20	5	na	na	na
A healthy choice, but probably high in sodium.						
Lo Mein Noodles—6 oz (Hibachi-San Japanese Grill)	270	42	6	1	na	690
A healthy choice.						
Beef Yakisoba—1 serving (Edo)	574	54	26	10	na	1122
High in fat and sodium.						
Hawaiian Chicken—1 serving (Edo)	500	71	8	2	na	716
A healthy choice.						
Veggie Bowl—1 (Teriyaki Stix)	440	95	1	0	na	880
High in carbs, low in fat, and high in sodium.						
Chicken Curry—1 serving (Teriyaki Stix)	650	92	17	6	na	1390
High in carbs, moderate in fat, and high in sodium.						
Teriyaki Chicken Salad—1 serving (Teriyaki Stix)	360	26	13	3	na	1320
A healthy choice other than the sodium count.						
Japanese Vegetable Teriyaki—1 dish (2½ servings) (Chin's Asia Fresh)	111	8	1	na	na	na
A healthy choice.						
Japanese Vegetable Teriyaki—1 serving (Chin's Asia Fresh)	45	8	1	na	na	na
A healthy choice.						

Menu Item	Calories	Carbohy-drate (g)	Fat (g)	Saturated Fat (g)	*Trans* Fat (g)	Sodium (mg)
Japanese Tofu Teriyaki—1 dish (2½ servings) (Chin's Asia Fresh)	226	17	13	na	na	na
A healthy choice.						
Japanese Tofu Teriyaki—1 dish (Chin's Asia Fresh)	90	7	5	na	na	na
A healthy choice.						
Tempura—3 Shrimp and Vegetables (www.calorieking.com)	320	25	18	na	na	na
The fat count is high because it's fried.						
Chicken Curry Bowl—1 serving (Teriyaki Stix)	660	92	17	6	na	1390
High in carbs, moderate in fat, and high in sodium.						
Ginger Pork—1 serving (Edo)	521	71	11	3	na	829
High in carbs, moderate in fat, and high in sodium.						
Grilled Vegetables—1 serving (Edo)	325	71	1	0	na	55
A healthy choice.						

The Menu Profile

Japanese cuisine focuses on the carbohydrates in rice, noodles, and vegetables and minimizes fats by using food preparation methods that require little or no oil or fat, such as steaming, braising, or simply serving it raw. Another big plus is that small portions are standard.

A number of healthy appetizers can be found on Japanese menus. Sushi and sashimi can be an appetizer or can make a whole meal. (Check the section "More About Sushi" on page 247 to learn more about sushi.) Beyond sushi, there are many other healthy appetizer choices, which is a rare delight because most appetizers in American and other style restaurants are fried and high in fat. Common hot appetizers are edamame, gyoza, and shumai, and cold appetizers include wakame and tofu. Some appetizers are partnered with a dipping sauce, but be careful when you use them—they are high in sodium. Avoid the few fried items—tempura, agetofu (fried bean curd), and fried dumplings.

Soup is a great, filling start to put a dent in your appetite or to order as an entrée. Light and delicate broth-based soups are widely available. Miso soup, which is mainly broth and bits of tofu and scallion, is the most commonly served soup. You may also choose a simple, clear broth called suimono, which has a base of dashi and bits of vegetables or meat. Udon, or dashi-based noodle soups, have a few more calories because of the noodles. Su-udon is plain broth with noodles. Other varieties of udon have stir-fried beef, vegetables, or tempura items added. Stick with the su-udon or yaki-udon.

You'll also find salads in Japanese restaurants that include tossed greens, tofu, seaweed, or seafood. In Japan, salads are called sunomono or aemono. They consist of vinegared or otherwise dressed vegetables and seafoods served in small quantities in elegant little bowls. On top, expect a light miso dressing.

Most Japanese entrées are low in fat and potentially low in saturated fat and cholesterol—if you choose wisely. Several styles of food preparation are usually stated on the menu. For example, chicken, beef, or salmon can be prepared teriyaki-style. The same goes for nabemonos, which are one-pot meals. Sukiyaki, yosenabi, and shabu-shabu are members of the nabemonos family.

Donburi is a rice dish topped with broiled or fried meat, fish, poultry, eggs, and soy sauce. Obviously, donburi is best topped with broiled items instead of breaded and fried ones. Because of the whole eggs it contains, donburi should be avoided by cholesterol watchers (or you can simply request that the egg be left off).

Sake is a fermented rice wine. It is typically served hot or cold in decanters and poured into very small cups. Sake's calories come mainly from alcohol; only a few come from carbohydrates. An ounce of sake contains about 40 calories; if it's a drink you enjoy, go ahead and indulge.

Japanese restaurants are not known for their desserts. You'll see a short list of desserts in most full-menu Japanese restaurants: fresh fruit, green-tea or red-bean ice cream, and perhaps yo kan, a sweet bean cake.

Japanese cuisine is relatively high in sodium because of its many soy-based items. Japanese marinades and sauces, including teriyaki, sukiyaki, or shabu-shabu, are a combination of some or all of the following ingredients: shoyu, dashi, mirin, sugar, sake, and kombu.

Ordering fish, shellfish, or poultry instead of beef or pork helps keep the fat down. Fortunately, portion size is usually far more consistent with healthy guidelines than most American meals. Like with other Asian cuisines, it's also easy to limit portion size by ordering family-style.

If fats are used in Japanese cooking, they are mainly the cholesterol-free varieties like cottonseed, olive, peanut, or sesame seed oil. Sesame seed oil is used in small quantities for its wonderful nutty flavor.

It is typical to see sugar in many Japanese food preparations, as is true with most Southeast Asian cuisines. Sugar is used in almost all the sauces and marinades. Sugar is also found in su, or "vinegared" rice, which is used in sushi. In the end, most sauces and dishes will not provide you with more than several teaspoons to a single tablespoon of sugar.

More about Sushi

Sushi and sashimi have a long heritage. Many different finfish, shellfish, eggs, and/or vegetables are used in its preparation.

Sushi began centuries ago as a method of preserving fish. At that time, sushi was rice that had been vinegared (mixed with sugar and vinegar) and placed either side of a piece of dried fish. Much later, a thin piece of nori, or seaweed, was added to make it easier to eat with your hands.

Sushi is served as rolls, as pieces of fish served atop a bed of sushi rice, or as hand rolls, cone-shaped pieces of seaweed in which rice, fish and/or other items are placed. People who are unfamiliar with sushi often think that it always contains raw fish, but that is not always the case. Cooked fish, such as crab, shrimp, surimi (imitation crab), soft-shell crab, eel, and others are often used in rolls. Fish-free (a.k.a. "vegetarian") sushi is also available, with vegetables like cucumber and avocado.

Su, or "vinegared," rice is flavored with vinegar, salt, and sugar. The blend of these ingredients gives it its sticky quality. The volume of rice used in sushi ranges. In general, the more expensive the sushi, the less rice is used. Expect to see more rice, wasabi, and ginger, and less fish in all-you-can-eat sushi restaurants.

Great importance is placed on the freshness of the fish and the creativity with which sushi is served. You should be smart about where you eat raw fish. Choose a reputable restaurant that serves a lot of sushi. Make sure the sushi chefs are working with clean hands. If the raw fish doesn't smell or look fresh to you, don't eat it and send it back.

For the most part, you can't go wrong with sushi and sashimi, but watch out for some of the Americanized types of sushi. The Philadelphia roll, which includes cream cheese, and tempura rolls, which include tempura-fried vegetables or seafood, should be skipped. Also, look out for mayonnaise-based sauces. Even if you do indulge in these choices, the small amounts of fat that these sushi types contain don't hold a candle to the amount of fat in a hamburger and fries.

▷ Green Flag Words

The asterisks (*) denote foods that are high in sodium.

Ingredients

△ clear broth

△ vinegared, seasoned, or su rice (vinegar, salt, and sugar added)

△ vinegar sauce*

△ soy sauce*

△ teriyaki sauce*

△ miso dressing*

△ dipping sauce*

△ udon, rice, or bean thread noodles

△ seafood (raw and cooked finfish and shellfish)

△ chicken

△ cucumber

△ avocado

△ spinach

△ tofu

△ soybeans (edamame)

Cooking Methods/Menu Descriptions/Names

△ steamed (mushimono)

△ sautéed

△ nabemono (one-pot meal)

△ braised

△ simmered (nimono)

△ marinated

△ pickled

△ raw
△ broiled (yaki)
△ barbecued
△ grilled (yakimono)
△ on skewers
△ boiled
△ served in broth*
△ with vegetables
△ salads

▶ Red Flag Words

Ingredients

▼ fried bean curd
▼ cream cheese
▼ mayonnaise-based sauces for sushi

Cooking Methods/Menu Descriptions/Names

▼ deep-fried, battered and fried, breaded and fried
▼ tempura
▼ agemono (deep fried)
▼ katsu (fried)
▼ pan-fried

At the Table

▼ soy sauce*

Special Requests

- "Could you serve the salad dressing on the side?"
- "I'm carefully watching my salt intake. Can you use less soy sauce when preparing this dish?"
- "Could you hold the salt on the edamame?"

- ◆ "Could you add cucumber to the eel and avocado sushi roll?"
- ◆ "Please don't use mayonnaise-based sauce on the sushi."
- ◆ "Could you substitute shrimp, scallops, or chicken for the beef in this dish?"
- ◆ "Could you leave the egg out of the donburi?"
- ◆ "I couldn't finish this. May I get it wrapped up to take home?"

Typical Menu: Japanese Style

✿ *Indicates preferred choices*

Sushi (served with wasabi, pickled ginger, and soy sauce)

- ✿ **Nigiri-sushi** (tuna, yellowtail, cooked shrimp, or salmon served on rice)
- ✿ **Maki-sushi** (eel and cucumber roll, California roll, tuna roll)
- ✿ **Temaki sushi** (hand rolls; crab and cucumber, spicy tuna, smoked salmon, avocado roll)
- ✿ **Futomaki** (thick rolls with vegetables, mushrooms, and egg)

Sashimi (served with wasabi, pickled ginger, and soy sauce)

- ✿ **Tuna**
- ✿ **Salmon**
- ✿ **Yellowtail**

Appetizers

- ✿ **Yutofu** (hot bean curd boiled with napa and served with special sauce)
- ✿ **Ebisu** (shrimp in vinegar sauce)

- ✲ **Edamame** (steamed and salted soybeans in their pods) (Note: Ask the server to hold the salt.)
- ✲ **Shumai** (steamed shrimp dumplings wrapped in thin noodle skin)
- **Tempura** appetizer (shrimp and vegetables dipped in batter and lightly fried)
- ✲ **Yakitori** (two skewers of chicken broiled with teriyaki sauce)
- **Agedashi tofu** (fried tofu in tempura sauce)
- ✲ **Ohitashi** (fresh spinach boiled and served with soy sauce)
- ✲ **Wakame** (dried seaweed marinated and served in long strands)
- ✲ **Gyoza** (pork dumplings and vegetable)

Soups

- ✲ **Suimono** (clear broth soup)
- ✲ **Miso** (soybean paste soup with tofu and scallions)
- ✲ **Su-udon** (plain Japanese noodle soup)
- **Tempura-udon** (Japanese noodle soup with tempura)
- ✲ **Yaki-udon** (Japanese noodle soup with stir-fried vegetables)

Salads

- ✲ **Tossed salad** (served with miso dressing)
- ✲ **Tofu salad** (served with miso dressing)
- ✲ **Seafood sunomono** (seafood with cucumber, seaweed, and shredded garnish with vinegar sauce)

Entrées (served à la carte with steamed white rice or soba noodles)

- **Tempura** (lightly battered and fried shrimp, vegetable, or a combination of the two served with tempura sauce)

✿ **Agemono** (pork cutlet, chicken, or shrimp battered in bread crumbs and deep-fried)

✿ **Teriyaki** (chicken, beef, or salmon broiled and served with teriyaki sauce)

✿ **Sukiyaki** (chicken or beef simmered in sukiyaki sauce with tofu, bamboo shoots, and vegetables)

✿ **Yosenabe** (noodles, seafood, and vegetables simmered in a special broth)

✿ **Shabu-shabu** (sliced beef and vegetables with noodles cooked and served with dipping sauces)

Donburi (sautéed chicken, egg, and onion; deep-fried breaded pork, egg, onion; or broiled eel served on a bed of rice with a special sauce)

Desserts

✿ **Fresh fruit**

Ice cream (ginger, red bean, green tea, or vanilla)

Yo kan (sweet bean cake)

·················· ◀ **"May I Take Your Order?"** ▶ ··················

Low-Calorie Sample Meal

Sashimi, tuna (raw tuna and su rice)
Quantity: 2 pieces
Maki-sushi (California roll)
Quantity: 4 pieces (crab, cucumber, avocado and su rice)
Soy sauce, wasabi, and pickled ginger for above
Yaki-udon soup
Quantity: 1½ cups
Tofu salad (dressing on the side)
Quantity: 1 cup
Miso dressing for above (on the side)
Quantity: 2 tablespoons

> **NUTRITION SUMMARY**
> 630 calories
> Carbohydrate: 85 g, 54%
> Fat: 13 g, 18%
> Protein: 44 g, 28%
> Cholesterol: 76 mg
> Sodium: 1490 mg

Moderate-Calorie Sample Meal

Ohitashi
Quantity: 1 order
Suimono soup
Quantity: 1 cup
Teriyaki, salmon (½ order)
Quantity: 4 oz.
Donburi, oyako (½ order)
Quantity: 1½ cups
Steamed rice
Quantity: ⅔ cup
Orange sections
Quantity: 2 quarters

> **NUTRITION SUMMARY**
> 720 calories
> Carbohydrate: 85 g, 47%
> Fat: 19 g, 23%
> Protein: 54 g, 30% calories
> Cholesterol: 251 mg (mainly from the egg in the donburi)
> Sodium: 1700 mg

Japanese Menu Lingo

Bonito: an important fish in Japanese cuisine, it is a member of the mackerel family; bonito flakes are an important ingredient in the basic stock (broth) dashi.

Daikon: a giant white radish; grated daikon is mixed into tempura sauces, sliced daikon can be used in sushi.

Dashi: an important element in Japanese cooking, dashi is the basic stock made with water, kombu (seaweed), and bonito flakes.

Edamame: steamed or boiled soybeans that are served warmed and salted.

Gynniku: beef.

Kombu: a Japanese seaweed central to the basic stock (broth) dashi that is also used in sauces and as a wrapper for certain dishes.

Mirin: a Japanese rice wine that is used more often in sauces than as a beverage. It is a central ingredient in the sauces and flavors of Japanese cuisine.

Miso: a fermented soybean paste that comes in various types, thicknesses, and degrees of saltiness. It is used in soups, sauces, and dressings and is a basic ingredient in Japanese cooking.

Nori: a seaweed that is often toasted prior to use. It has a strong flavor and is used to wrap maki sushi (both rolls and hand rolls).

Sake: fermented rice wine, sake is the national alcoholic beverage of Japan. It is usually served warm and is also used as an ingredient in sauces.

Shiitake: an abundant mushroom in Japanese food, it has a woody and fruity flavor. It is used fresh or dried.

Shoyu: Japanese soy sauce, which comes in light and dark varieties. It is made from soybeans, wheat, and salt, and is an essential ingredient in Japanese cooking.

Teriyaki sauce: a sauce used to broil that is made with shoyu and mirin. Teriyaki means "shining broil."

Tofu soybean curd: a major source of protein in the Japanese diet that is used in soups, appetizers, salads, and entrées.

Ton: pork.

Tori: chicken.

Vinegar: in Japan, it is made from rice and is lighter and sweeter than the vinegar Americans are used to.

Wakame: a seaweed used for its flavor and texture that is available dried.

Wasabi: called Japanese horseradish, it is fragrant and sharp in taste and is regularly served with sushi and sashimi.

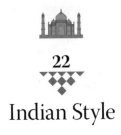

22

Indian Style

India's location tells a lot about the distinctive flavors of its cuisines. Indian food closely resembles the cuisines of its neighbors—Pakistan, Sri Lanka, Thailand, China, and Burma. However, Indian food is most similar to that of Thailand, in terms of its spices and ingredients. The dishes of both countries can be hot and spicy, employ the spices that combine to make curry, and are often accompanied by rice (however, flavorful steamed white basmati rice is the type most commonly served in Indian restaurants).

India is one of the world's largest and most populous countries. Regional cuisines have developed because of the vast size of the country and because its different areas produce different foods and ingredients. Northern Indian food is considerably cooler to the taste buds than southern Indian cuisine, which makes abundant use of chilies and peppers. The north uses more wheat products, teas, and eggs, and the south features more rice, vegetables, and coffee. More seafood is eaten in the south, which abuts the sea, but yogurt is a common ingredient used in both northern and southern Indian cooking. Most Indian restaurants in America feature northern cuisine.

The influx of Indian emigres in the U.S. has increased greatly over the last several decades. As is true for most migrations of people, their foods, and their ways of serving it, have come along too. Today, Indian restaurants are quite common in the United States, particularly in middle- to large-size metropolitan areas. Most Indian restaurants are sit-down establishments and are independently owned and operated. One owner might own just one or a few restaurants. There are no large chains that feature Indian food, and only a few independent restaurants offer Indian fast food.

Dishes you can expect to find on Indian menus in America include the appetizers samosa and pakora; the entrées tandoori chicken, chicken vindaloo, and vegetable curry; and the accompaniments mango chutney and raita. Eating healthy is easier than in many American-style restaurants. For starters, portions are smaller. Indian meals also feature many vegetables and legumes (chickpeas) and flavor the foods with nonfat herbs, spices, and other seasonings. The key challenge is limiting fried foods and overuse of butter, which is called ghee.

The Menu Profile

As with most ethnic cuisines, there are health pros and cons to Indian cooking. If you have some basic knowledge of the cuisine, are careful about reading the food descriptions, and ask a lot of questions, you'll have no problem. For help with menu lingo, consult the glossary at the end of this chapter.

The pros include the accent on starches and vegetables (carbohydrates) and lack of emphasis on meats (protein). Basmati rice, the premier flavorful rice, is a main element of Indian cuisine. Breads are also considered an important and regular element of the meal—but diners need to be careful about the fried breads. Legumes, including lentils and chickpeas, are often found in dishes or accompaniments; they are good sources of soluble fiber and nonanimal protein. Vegetables are a primary part of most meals, including curry dishes, biryani (rice dishes), and pullao (basmati rice served with entrées). Commonly served vegetables include spinach, eggplant, cabbage, potatoes, and peas, and onions, green peppers, and tomatoes are often found in stewed entrées. Plain yogurt is frequently used in sauces.

Another positive aspect of Indian cuisine that helps you keep protein, calories, and cholesterol low is the predominance of chicken and seafood. Beef and lamb are found on the menus, too, but there are so many delicious poultry and fish options that you probably won't be tempted to go with red meat. Pork and pork products are rarely found on Indian menus. Small quantities of protein are used, and it's easy to eat vegetarian if you desire. If two people share a chicken or shrimp masala, each person won't have more than two to three ounces of protein—just the right amount. It's wise for a party of four to order one chicken or seafood dish and one vegetable dish (maybe a biryani or aloo chole) to keep the calories, protein, and fat low.

Garam masala, which is a fragrant mix of ground spices, produces many of the wonderful tastes of Indian cuisine. The "C" spices found in garam masala are cardamom, coriander, cumin, cloves, and cinnamon. Several of these spices are referred to as "fragrant" spices. Southern Indian cuisine adds pepper and chilies to the mix to raise the "heat." Mint, garlic, ginger, plain yogurt, and coconut milk are other common ingredients in Indian cooking. Find more of these spices and ingredients defined in the section "Indian Menu Lingo" at the end of this chapter.

Probably the most negative aspect of Indian cuisine is its high fat content. Ghee, which is clarified butter, is a common ingredient used in food preparation. Frying and sautéing are common preparation methods. For example, most appetizers, such as samosa and pakora, are fried. Some breads, such as paratha and poori, are deep fried, and others are brushed with oil or butter.

The oils most frequently used in Indian cooking are sesame

and coconut oil. Sesame oil is primarily a polyunsaturated oil, but coconut oil is about the most saturated oil there is. Ask your server what kind of oil the restaurant uses; if it is coconut oil, avoid the fried foods altogether.

As with Thai food, coconut milk is used in Indian cooking, especially in soups and curry dishes. Coconut milk contributes calories, fat, and saturated fat. Look for the words coconut milk, coconut cream, or shredded coconut in menu descriptions and avoid items that contain them.

The sodium content of an Indian meal can be kept within bounds by navigating around the menu carefully. In particular, Indian soups tend to be high in sodium, so it is best to avoid them if you are watching your sodium levels closely. Many dishes have small amounts of salt added, but if it is divided into a number of servings and you keep the portions small, your consumption will be minimal.

A healthy appetizer is a rarity: Samosas are fried turnovers stuffed with peas and potatoes; cheese, chicken, or vegetable pakoras are all fried; and shrimp with poori is fried as well. If you can find them, chicken tikha kabobs are a healthy choice. One item that serves as an appetizer, a condiment, and a bread is papadum, a thin wafer made from spicy lentils. If you can handle the hot taste, papadum is baked and is the best of the appetizer choices. If you have calories to spare, share one appetizer with a dining companion. If you're with a group that orders several appetizers or a combination plate (consider it an Indian-style poo-poo platter), decide which item is the healthiest and take one piece.

You may choose mulligatawny or lentil soup as a meal starter (again, if you are not closely watching your sodium intake). They are both seasoned with Indian spices, are quite tasty, contain healthy legumes, and are low in fat and calories. Creamy soups, such as poppy seed and coconut, should be avoided.

Ordering bread can present some difficulties, but there are several healthy choices. Papadum, which may also be called papad, is a crisp, spicy, baked lentil wafer. Chapati is a flat disk of unleavened bread that resembles pita bread; it is sometimes made with whole-wheat flour. Nan is a leavened bread that is made with white flour and available plain or seasoned with garlic or stuffed with cheese or meat. (Stick with the plain or garlic varieties.) There are three other options as well: kulcha, a baked bread stuffed with vegetables such as onions; roti, a bread made with whole-wheat flour and baked; and pratha, a multilayered unleavened bread that is sometimes prepared with whole-wheat flour. Always request that the bread not be topped with ghee (butter) or oil. Poori, a light, puffed fried bread should be skipped.

Moving on to the entrées. You'll find that similar cooking styles are used for chicken, fish, shrimp, beef, and lamb dishes. To keep total fat, saturated fat, and calories down, stick with fish, chicken, or shrimp prepared in the following styles: masala, a combination of Indian spices with sautéed tomatoes and onions; bhuna, a similar preparation to masala; jalpharezi, which is cooked with vegetables; saag, which has spinach and spices; matar, which is cooked with green peas; and vindaloo, a mixture of Indian spices with potatoes. Tandoori and tikka dishes are another healthy option; they are prepared in a clay oven, which is called a tandoor. Avoid malai and korma dishes, which are creamy.

In most restaurants, you'll probably be served plain pullao (basmati rice touched with saffron) with your entrée. If you want more rice, choose a biryani. Biryanis, which can contain chicken, lamb, beef, shrimp, or vegetables, are listed under rice dishes but can be excellent high-carbohydrate, low-protein entrées. A chicken masala can be a very nice complement to a shrimp biryani if you can share with a dining companion. If you do choose to share, ask your server to skip the pullao with the masala, as that would be too much rice.

Vegetable dishes can easily be a main course as long as you skip the fried choices. Vegetable dishes use a variety of chickpeas, lentils, potatoes, spinach, cauliflower, onions, and/or tomatoes in curry or cheese (paneer) sauces. Paneer, which is the most commonly used form of cheese in Indian cookery, is not like cheese in America. Paneer is an unaged non-melting cheese, like farmer cheese. It is made from milk and set (formed into blocks) with an acid—usually lemon juice. Paneer has an added bonus: No salt is added in its preparation process.

A fun and unique part of Indian cuisine are its accompaniments. Raita, a combination of plain yogurt, cucumbers, and onions (and sometimes tomatoes or fruit), is quite healthy and cools the mouth after you consume hot curries. Dal is a lowfat, spicy, lentil-based side sauce that is served warm. Onion chutney, which may also be called relish, may also be placed on your table. It is quite low in calories and adds zip. Other chutneys, such as mint and tamarind, are also low in calories. Mango chutney, which is quite sweet and contains small pieces of mango and sugar, is very popular in U.S. Indian restaurants and is relatively high in calories. You'll also find pickles prepared with a variety of low-calorie ingredients and hot spices. Accompaniments are eaten in very small quantities and most are quite low in fat, so feel free to indulge in them when eating Indian food.

▷ Green Flag Words

Ingredients

- △ skinless chicken
- △ shrimp and other seafood (not fried)
- △ baked leavened bread made with whole wheat flour
- △ papadum

△ vegetables—tomatoes, onions, spinach, and potatoes

△ ginger and garlic

△ nuts

△ dried fruit

△ lentils, chickpeas and peas (matta)

△ potatoes

△ Indian spices and combinations—curry, garam masala, saffron

△ basmati rice (pullao)

Cooking Methods/Menu Descriptions/Names

△ tikka

△ tandoori

△ cooked with or marinated in yogurt

△ cooked with onions, tomatoes, spinach, peppers, potatoes, or peas

△ masala

△ paneer (homemade cheese)

△ marinated or cooked in Indian spices

△ Indian hot spices

△ garnished with dried fruits

△ chutneys—mango, mint

△ pickle

△ raita

△ dal (lentils)

△ kebab

▶ Red Flag Words

Ingredients

▼ ghee

▼ molee (coconut)

▼ coconut milk

Cooking Methods/Menu Descriptions/Names

- ▾ fritters
- ▾ fried, deep-fried
- ▾ dipped in batter, chickpea batter
- ▾ korma (cream sauce)
- ▾ stuffed and fried
- ▾ sautéed in butter, served in butter sauce
- ▾ creamy curry sauce

Special Requests

- ◆ "Please bring the accompaniments raita, dal, and onion chutney."
- ◆ "Since we are also having a biryani, please do not bring the plain pullao with our other dish."
- ◆ "My order will be à la carte and not a complete dinner."
- ◆ "Can you prepare this dish with chicken instead of lamb?"
- ◆ "Can my dish be prepared without adding any salt?"
- ◆ "Please bring my salad (or soup) when the others have their appetizers."
- ◆ "Can you please make sure that no ghee is placed on my bread?"
- ◆ "I'll have tea (or water) as my beverage."

Typical Menu: Indian Style

✿ *Indicates preferred choices*

Appetizers

Cheese pakoras (homemade cheese deep-fried in a chickpea batter)
Vegetable pakoras (assorted vegetables formed into fritters and deep-fried in a chickpea batter)

Samosa (a vegetable turnover, stuffed and fried)

☼ **Chicken tikha** (pieces of chicken roasted with herbs on skewers in a tandoor oven)

Fried shrimp with poori (shrimp with onions and peppers fried with spices)

☼ **Papadum, or papad** (crispy, thin lentil wafers)

Soups

☼ **Mulligatawny** (lentils, vegetables, and spices)

Coconut soup (coconut cream and pistachio nuts)

☼ **Dal rasam** (pepper soup with lentils)

Breads (Roti)

Paratha (multilayered bread made with butter; ask your server to hold the butter)

Poori (light, puffed fried bread)

☼ **Chapati** (thin, dry whole-wheat bread)

☼ **Nan** (leavened baked bread, plain or with onions)

☼ **Onion Kulcha** (unleavened bread stuffed with onions)

☼ **Aloo Kulcha** (unleavened bread stuffed with spiced potatoes)

Chicken (Murgi)

☼ **Chicken tandoori** (chicken marinated in spices and roasted in a tandoor oven)

☼ **Chicken tikka** (chicken roasted in charcoal oven with mild spices)

☼ **Chicken vindaloo** (boneless chicken cooked with potatoes and hot spices)

Chicken kandhari (chicken cooked with cream sauce and cashews)

☼ **Chicken masala** (roasted chicken cooked in spices and a thick curry sauce)

Shrimp/Fish

Shrimp malai (shrimp cooked with cream, mushrooms, and coconut)

✿ **Shrimp bhuna** (shrimp cooked with green vegetables, onions, and tomatoes)

✿ **Fish masala** (boneless fish marinated in a spicy yogurt sauce)

Shrimp curry (shrimp cooked in a thick curry sauce)

✿ **Shrimp vindaloo** (shrimp cooked with potatoes in a hot curry sauce)

Beef/Lamb

✿ **Lamb bhuna** (lamb pan-roasted with spices, onions, and tomatoes)

✿ **Lamb saag** (lamb cooked with spinach in a spicy curry sauce)

✿ **Beef vindaloo** (beef cooked with potatoes in a hot curry sauce)

Beef korma (beef curry cooked with cream)

Rice (pullao)

✿ **Shrimp biryani** (shrimp cooked with basmati rice)

✿ **Vegetable biryani** (basmati rice cooked with green vegetables)

✿ **Plain pullao** (basmati rice cooked with saffron)

✿ **Peas pullao** (basmati rice cooked with peas)

Vegetables

✿ **Vegetable curry** (green peas, tomatoes, and cauliflower cooked in a curry sauce)

Vegetable korma (mixed vegetables cooked with cream, herbs, and cashews)

- ☼ **Saag paneer** (spinach cooked with homemade cheese)
- ☼ **Aloo chole** (chickpeas cooked with tomatoes and potatoes)

Accompaniments

- ☼ **Raita** (yogurt with grated cucumbers, onions, and spices)
- ☼ **Mint chutney**
- ☼ **Mango chutney** (Note: Mango chutney is high in carbohydrate and sugar, and relatively high in calories.)
- ☼ **Onion chutney** (diced onions with hot spices)
- ☼ **Dal** (lentil-based sauce)
- ☼ **Tamata salat** (diced tomatoes and onions with hot spices and lemon)

Desserts

Koulfi (a rich ice cream with almonds and pistachios)
Gulab jamun (fried milk balls soaked in sugar syrup, served warm)
Ras malai (homemade cheese in sweetened milk)

.... ◀ **"May I Take Your Order?"** ▶ ....

Low-Calorie Sample Meal

Nan
Quantity: ¼ loaf
Shrimp biryani
Quantity: 1 cup
Raita
Quantity: 3 tablespoons
Onion chutney
Quantity: 2 tablespoons
Tamata salat
Quantity: ½ cup
Darjeeling tea
Quantity: 2 cups

> **NUTRITION SUMMARY**
> 480 calories
> Carbohydrate: 60 g, 50%
> Fat: 13 g, 25%
> Protein: 29 g, 24%
> Cholesterol: 128 mg
> Sodium: 950 mg

Moderate-Calorie Sample Meal

Samosa
Quantity: 1 piece
Chicken tandoori
Quantity: 4 oz. (½ order)
Peas pullao
Quantity: 1 cup
Saag paneer
Quantity: 1 cup
Mint chutney
Quantity: 2 tablespoons
Dal
Quantity: 3 tablespoons

> **NUTRITION SUMMARY**
> 850 calories
> Carbohydrate: 83 g, 39%
> Fat: 36 g, 38%
> Protein: 49 g, 23%
> Cholesterol: 93 mg
> Sodium: 1700 mg

Indian Menu Lingo

Bombay duck: actually not duck at all, it is fish served either sautéed, fried, or dried alongside with curry and rice. It is relatively uncommon on U.S. Indian restaurant menus.

Cardamom: an expensive spice native to India that is from the ginger family. Either the whole cardamom pod or only seeds are used. It is one of the most common spices found in garam masalas (curry mixtures).

Cinnamon: a delicate spice commonly found in curries and spice combinations. Stick cinnamon, which has more intense flavor, is used in Indian cooking, and ground cinnamon, which is commonly used in the U.S., is rarely used in Indian cooking.

Clove: another commonly used spice in curries that is the dried flower bud of an evergreen tropical tree found in Southeast Asia.

Coconut milk: a creamy fluid extracted from coconut flesh.

Coriander: a fragrant spice that is often the main ingredient in curries. Either ground coriander or the whole leaf (which is also known as cilantro) is used. Also called Chinese parsley.

Cumin: a fragrant spice important to curry dishes that is used as seeds or ground.

Curry: "curry" is not an individual spice used in Indian cooking. The word means "sauce," and many individually roasted spices make up a curry mixture known as *garam masala*.

Fennel: a spice used in curries that is a member of the cumin family and is occasionally referred to as sweet cumin.

Ghee: clarified butter that contains no milk solids.

Malai: a thick cream made by separating and collecting the top part of boiled milk; used in entrées for a thick, creamy sauce.

Mint: an herb used to add flavor to curry dishes and also as a main ingredient in mint chutney and mint sambal. It is also used in biryani and in dipping sauces for appetizers.

Paneer: referred to as homemade cream cheese or cottage cheese, it is made by curdling milk with lemon juice and straining it through cheesecloth. Paneer is used in vegetable and rice dishes, and for vegetarians, it is a complete protein source.

Poppy seeds: seeds that are ground into a powder and used to thicken the sauces in curry dishes.

Rose water: a flavoring agent used in Indian desserts made by diluting the essence of rose petals.

Saffron: widely known as the most expensive spice in the world, it is obtained by drying the stamens of saffron crocus flowers. Small quantities are used commonly in Indian cooking.

Tamarind: a fruit from a large tropical tree that is used for its acidic quality, it is commonly used in Indian food.

Turmeric: a spice that lends a yellow-orange color to commercial curry powder. It is a member of the ginger family and is commonly used in Indian cooking.

Yogurt: a common ingredient in Indian cooking that is always plain and unflavored.

23

Middle Eastern Style

Referring to all Middle Eastern restaurants as belonging to a single cuisine doesn't do justice to the individualities of the cuisines from this region of the world. Yes, there are similarities between the cuisines of Middle Eastern countries, including Greece, Lebanon, Turkey, Israel, Iran, Morocco, Syria, and many more. But there are also unique qualities of each cuisine. The most common Middle Eastern cuisine in the U.S. is Greek, but as more people from other Middle Eastern nations emigrate to the U.S., other choices will gain in popularity.

The geographic locale of the Middle Eastern countries has a large impact on the ingredients and spices used and the flavors of the cuisine. Commonly used spices include parsley, mint, cilantro, and oregano, plus a host of others that are also mainstays in Indian cooking—cumin, coriander, cinnamon, and ginger. Long ago, the Middle East was a critical link on the spice route between the Far East and Europe.

Middle Eastern restaurants range from mall eateries that confine their menus to gyros and souvlaki sandwiches to upscale white-tablecloth dinner spots that serve more traditional fare. Some of these restaurants specialize in one Middle Eastern cuisine in particular. You'll also find some Middle Eastern foods integrated into "American" restaurant menus; for example, it's common to see gyros and Greek salads on the menus of sandwich shops or family-fare restaurants. Several Middle Eastern foods, such as hummus, baba ghanoush, and feta cheese, are stocked in just about every supermarket.

Nutrition Snapshot

The following nutrition snapshot is intended to provide you with the nutrition numbers for a handful of common menu items served at Middle Eastern restaurants. Unfortunately, there is little nutrition data available for Middle Eastern restaurant foods, because most Middle Eastern restaurants are independently owned. Because it's common to see a scattering of Middle Eastern items for sale in supermarkets, reviewing the nutrition facts from these foods can also provide you some insight. Use this data to educate yourself about the nutrition facts of your Middle Eastern favorites. If necessary, make changes to eat healthier.

Menu Item	Calories	Carbohydrate (g)	Fat (g)	Saturated Fat (g)	*Trans* Fat (g)	Sodium (mg)
Hummus (2 tbsp.) (USDA data)	53	6	3	0	na	73
A healthy bet for dipping. The creamier and lighter in color the hummus, the more high-fat tahini is likely added. Ask your server not to add any extra oil.						
Baba Ghanoush (2 tbsp.) (www.calorieking.com)	70	1	3	na	na	na
A healthy bet for dipping. Ask your server not to add any extra oil.						
Pita Bread (1 6½" piece) (USDA data)	165	33	1	0	na	322
A lowfat choice.						
Grape Leaves Stuffed with Rice (0.9 oz. per single grape leaf) (www.calorieking.com)	35	6	1	0	na	60
Have a few. They are healthy.						
Falafel (1 2¼") (USDA data for home-prepared)	57	5	3	0	na	50
They are usually fried, but they are still a healthy choice because they are made from garbanzo beans.						

Menu Item	Calories	Carbohy-drate (g)	Fat (g)	Saturated Fat (g)	*Trans* Fat (g)	Sodium (mg)
Falafel (1 serving/2.8 oz) (USDA data)	253	27	13	0	na	27
They are usually fried, but they are still a healthy choice because they are made from garbanzo beans.						
Spinach Pie (3½ oz.) (www.calorieking.com)	290	20	21	na	na	na
Skip it. The spinach is smothered in high-fat phyllo and feta cheese surrounds.						
Feta Cheese (1 oz.) (USDA data)	75	1	6	4	na	316
One of the healthier cheeses, but still high in fat and saturated fat.						
Beef Shawarma (Rotisserie-Cooked Beef) (4 oz.) (www.calorieking.com)	280	2	15	na	na	na
Choose the chicken shawarma instead of beef to cut the fat grams.						
Fried Kibbeh (3 oz.) (www.calorieking.com)	180	15	8	na	na	na
Not bad for fried, but this is a small portion.						
Greek Salad (11.5 oz.) (Atlanta Bread Company) (no dressing)	200	13	13	6	na	na
Feta cheese is the high-fat ingredient. If made to order ask them to go light on the feta.						
Greek Salad Dressing (2 tbsp.) (Atlanta Bread Company)	100	1	10	2	na	420
Pour the salad dressing gingerly.						
Tahini (Sesame Seed Paste) (1 tbsp.) (www.calorieking.com)	90	2	8	na	na	na
Loaded with fat. Use sparingly.						
Labneh (~ 2 oz.) (www.calorieking.com)	70	4	2	2	na	100
Yogurt-based sauce for sandwiches that really beats mayonnaise.						
Baklava (~ 2 oz.) (www.calorieking.com)	245	18	18	na	na	na
Fat and calories are high. Enjoy no more than a nibble or two.						

*The nutrition information for many of these items is based on commercially prepared and supermarket available foods. Foods prepared in restaurants may differ in their nutrient composition.

The Menu Profile

As usual, the foods that play a predominant role in Middle Eastern cooking are those that are naturally plentiful in the region—wheat, grains, legumes, olives, dates, figs, lamb, and eggplant, to name a few.

Rice combined with a variety of ingredients to make rice pilaf is commonly served in Greece and the Middle East, and cous-cous, which is made with cracked wheat, is indigenous to North African countries. Tabouli, the cold cracked wheat or bulgur salad tossed with raw vegetables and lots of parsley, is a key part of Lebanese cuisine, but it is commonly found throughout the Middle East.

Pita bread or pockets, as they're called in America, are flat, round breads that are only slightly leavened. Because they are cooked in a very hot oven, the resulting steam causes the bread to have a hollow center. This "pocket" is perfect for stuffing. Although whole-wheat pita breads are available in most super-markets, the pita bread served in restaurants is usually made with white flour.

It is common to find stuffed dishes. Probably the best known is dolma, which are stuffed grape leaves, but you will also find stuffed cabbage and eggplant. The stuffings are usually meat, rice, or vegetarian mixtures.

Chickpeas, fava beans, and other legumes are indigenous to the Middle East. Chickpeas and fava beans are puréed together to make falafel or ta'amia, and chickpeas are mashed and mixed with tahini (sesame seed paste or purée) to make hummus.

Because olives are so plentiful in the region, olive oil is the fat of choice. It is often used in cold dishes. Of course, it is good news that olive oil is used instead of butter (since is a mono-unsaturated fat), but remember—there are just as many calories in olive oil as there are in equal amounts of butter. Learn more about olives and olive oil in Chapter 17: Italian Style.

Lamb is the most common meat, and beef is also served, but to a lesser degree. Eggs are used quite a bit.

Milk is not a common ingredient in the Middle East because people of the region are frequently lactose intolerant, but plain yogurt is used in many dishes and sauces. For example, it is mixed with cucumber, garlic, mint, and/or salt to make tzatziki sauce, which is served as a side dish or used as a dressing for gyros and other kinds of sandwiches. Yogurt can also be used as a dressing for salads and in soups.

Feta and kasseri cheese are commonly used in Middle Eastern cookery. They may be served alone in chunks or incorporated into appetizers, salads, and entrées, such as Greek salad.

Phyllo (also filo or fila), which literally means leaf, is a paper-thin Middle Eastern dough. It is used to make sweet desserts, such as baklava, and dinner pies, such as spanakopita, the well-known spinach and feta cheese dish.

The appetizers, or mezza, as they may be called, are traditionally eaten leisurely. Several appetizers are high in fat and best limited: spanakopita, falafel (which is usually deep-fried), taramosalata, and cheese casserole. Baba ghanoush and hummus contain tahini (sesame seed paste), which boosts the fat, but it's healthy fat. You'll find baba ghanoush and hummus served with pita bread. Small amounts of these dishes are fine.

Better yet, hop over the appetizers and move directly to the salads. Greek or house salads are lettuce-based with cucumbers, tomatoes, onion, and a few high-sodium ingredients like cheese and olives. Don't forget to order your dressing on the side. You also might find fattoush, which is cucumbers, tomatoes, onions, and toasted pieces of pita bread. It might be predressed, because it usually marinates for a while. Tabouli, the cracked wheat salad, and tomato and cucumber salad are also regulars and very healthy—unless they are doused in oil or tahini.

A few soups are common on Middle Eastern menus. Lemon-egg soup (avgolemono) is a light and relatively low-calorie choice, but it does contain a fair amount of cholesterol. You might find a lentil, vegetable, or yogurt-based soup on the menu, all of which would be quite healthy.

When it comes to entrées, there's plenty of options. It's easy to order seafood or to go vegetarian, but beef and lamb are the predominant sources of protein. One choice is kibbeh, which is meat and cracked wheat with vegetables and spices tossed in; another is kafta, which is ground beef with onions, parsley, and spices. It's also easy to go vegetarian when ordering Middle Eastern food. Order stuffed eggplant or an appetizer and several à la carte salads. Grilling, stove-top cooking, and baking are the preparation methods of choice.

A very familiar entrée is shish kebab. Its origins relate to the time when the Ottoman armies camped outdoors and had to cook quickly. They devised the method of putting chunks of meat and vegetables on skewers and cooking them quickly over an open outdoor oven. Today, they are cooked on a grill. In most restaurants, you can order shish kebab with lamb, beef, chicken, or shrimp, and a combination is sometimes available. The meats are marinated in olive oil, lemon, wine, and spices and then grilled on a skewer with vegetables.

Eggplant is an ingredient used in several dishes. Moussaka, an eggplant and tomato sauce casserole with a white sauce topping, and sheikh el mahshi, which is stuffed eggplant with meat, are two common menu items. You should know that eggplant absorbs a lot of oil, and it is sometimes salted to remove its bitter taste. Avoid moussaka in particular because of the high fat content of its white sauce.

Gyros meat, a spicy combination of lamb and beef, and souvlaki, which is lamb, are often available wrapped in pita bread or served on platters. Both usually come with lettuce, tomato, onion, and tzatziki sauce. Tzatziki may be made with either with sour cream or yogurt. Always ask the restaurant whether low-calorie yogurt or high-fat sour cream is used as the base of its tzatziki sauce. Gyros and souvlaki are good choices, but try to eat more bread and vegetables than meat.

Lah me june is the Armenian answer to pizza. It's dough that is topped with ground meat, parsley, tomatoes, onions, and Middle Eastern spices. This is a good choice because it's low in protein and high in carbs. Omelettes made with feta cheese or lokaniko (sausage) and three eggs are offered on Middle Eastern menus. These are best avoided. Adding cheese or sauce to three eggs is enough cholesterol for several days—not to mention the fat.

Dinners in Middle Eastern restaurants are usually served with a small salad, pita bread, rice pilaf, and/or a steamed vegetable. All of these are relatively lowfat additions to a meal. If you closely watch your calories, pick and choose. Obviously, the salad and pita bread are great. When you order, don't feel compelled to include an entrée. Unless you can split or complement two dishes by sharing, that might be too much food and a setup to overeat.

Order à la carte appetizers, salads, and side dishes to create a healthy meal and taste more foods. Complement a few great-tasting and healthy appetizers with a healthy Greek salad. Create your own tapas. Another approach is to split everything with a partner, from appetizer to dessert: hummus and pita, lentil soup, couscous with lamb stew, and rice pudding. Or eat family style and order and divide a number of dishes. As always, order fewer dishes than there are people at the table, or be ready to store some food away as leftovers.

Dessert in the Middle East is traditionally just a bowl of fruit, but not so in Middle Eastern restaurants in America. You'll have the sweet choices of baklava, kataif, and rice pudding. Baklava is traditionally made with phyllo dough, plenty of butter, walnuts, sugar, and spices. A number of other varieties of baklava may be available that are prepared with different nuts and seasonings. Regardless, it's always high in fat and sugar. A few bites should be enough to satisfy your sweet tooth for a week or so.

Instead of indulging in one of these desserts, help yourself to a cup of Turkish or Greek coffee, which is served like espresso in Italian restaurants and upscale dining establishments. It is strong and sometimes thick or muddy, and it is served in small portions in demitasse cups. The coffee is delicious and has next to no calories.

▷ Green Flag Words

Ingredients

- △ lemon juice
- △ herbs and spices
- △ mint, parsley, onions, and cucumber
- △ mashed chickpeas
- △ fava beans
- △ eggplant
- △ with tomatoes, onions, and green peppers
- △ green beans, spinach
- △ grape leaves
- △ spiced ground beef or lamb
- △ gyro meat
- △ souvlaki
- △ cracked wheat (tabouli)
- △ pine nuts

△ olives

△ shrimp, squid (calamari)

△ yogurt

Cooking Methods/Menu Descriptions/Names

△ lemon dressing

△ tomato sauce

△ stuffed with ground lamb or meat

△ stuffed with rice and meat

△ grilled on a skewer (kebab)

△ marinated and barbecued

△ charcoal broiled

△ stewed

△ simmered

△ baked

△ dolmas, dolmatis

▶ Red Flag Words

* High in sodium and fat
+ High in sodium and cholesterol

Ingredients

▼ caviar*+

▼ tahini (ground sesame seeds)

▼ sesame seed paste or purée

▼ olive oil

▼ egg

▼ kalamata olives*

▼ Greek olives*

▼ feta cheese*

▼ kasseri cheese*

▼ lokaniko*

Cooking Methods/Menu Descriptions/Names

- ▼ phyllo dough
- ▼ foods made with tarator sauce
- ▼ lemon and butter sauce
- ▼ cheese pie
- ▼ spanikopita
- ▼ topped with creamy sauce
- ▼ béchamel sauce (white sauce)
- ▼ in pastry crust
- ▼ pan fried
- ▼ golden fried

Special Requests

- ◆ "Please bring my salad dressing on the side."
- ◆ "Please serve the tzatziki, salad dressing, or sauce for sandwiches on the side."
- ◆ "Please bring my salad (or soup) when you bring appetizers for the others."
- ◆ "Can I get olive oil and vinegar for my salad instead of the salad dressing?"
- ◆ "I'll have the appetizer portion, but serve it when you bring the others their entrées."
- ◆ "We're going to enjoy a Greek salad and share a few appetizers."
- ◆ "Can you leave the feta cheese and/or olives off the salad? I'm watching my sodium consumption."
- ◆ "Can please not add olive oil to the hummus, lebneh, or baba ghanoush?"
- ◆ "Please bring extra plates, because we're going to share."
- ◆ "Could I get a doggie bag when you bring the entrées? I'd like to put half away for tomorrow."

Typical Menu: Middle Eastern Style

✿ *Indicates preferred choices*

Appetizers

✿ **Hummus bi tahini** with pita bread (mashed chickpeas blended with tahini, lemon juice, and spices) (Note: Ask that the hummus not be topped with olive oil when it is served.)

✿ **Baba ghanoush** with pita bread (smoked eggplant mashed and combined with tahini, lemon juice, garlic, and other spices)

Taramosalata with pita bread (caviar blended with lemon juice and olive oil)

Kasseri casserole (kasseri cheese fried with a lemon and butter sauce)

Spanikopita (spinach and feta cheese pie made with phyllo dough)

✿ **Dolma** (cold grape leaves stuffed with a spicy combination of rice, onions, and tomatoes)

✿ **Ful Medames** (fava beans and chickpeas blended with spices and seasonings)

Falafel (a blend of chickpeas and fava beans, fried and served with tarator or tahini)

Salads

✿ **Greek salad** (lettuce, tomato, cucumbers, onions, feta cheese, and olives served with a light lemon and olive oil dressing)

✿ **Tabouli** (cracked wheat combined with parsley, tomatoes, cucumbers, lemon, and a spicy dressing)

✿ **Fattoush** (lettuce, peppers, scallions, onions, tomatoes, and pieces of toasted pita bread tossed and served with a light garlic and lemon dressing)

☼ **Yogurt salad** (yogurt mixed with fresh cucumber, garlic and mint) (Note: This salad may also be referred to as lebneh or tzatziki.)

Soups

☼ **Lentil soup** (lentils simmered with zucchini, celery, onions, potatoes, and spices)

☼ **Avgolemono** (a chicken broth-based soup with egg and lemon)

Entrées

☼ **Shish kebab** (chunks of marinated and spiced beef, lamb, or chicken skewered with tomatoes, onions, and peppers, and grilled)

Moussaka (layers of eggplant, ground lamb, and cheese topped with béchamel sauce)

Spanikopita (a spinach and cheese pie made with phyllo dough)

☼ **Kibbeh**, baked (cracked wheat mixed with spicy ground meat and sautéed onions and pine nuts)

☼ **Gyros** (a combination of seared spicy lamb and beef served with lettuce, tomato, onions, and tzatziki sauce)

☼ **Sheik el Mahshi** (baked eggplant stuffed with ground lamb, pine nuts, onions, Middle Eastern spices, and tomato sauce)

☼ **Souvlaki** (marinated and grilled beef or chicken served with lettuce, tomato, onions, and tzatziki sauce)

Pasticchio (baked macaroni with ground beef and eggs topped with a creamy sauce)

☼ **Dolma** (grape leaves, stuffed with ground lamb, rice, onions, and spices)

Falafel (fava beans and chickpeas blended with spices and served with tahini or tarator sauce)

✿ **Lah me june** (Armenian pizza topped with ground meat, parsley, tomatoes, onions, and spices)

✿ **Kafta** (grilled beef ground with parsley, onions, and other spices)

Side Dishes

✿ **Tabouli** (bulgur salad with raw vegetables)

✿ **Couscous** (a wheat grain steamed in a spicy lamb and vegetable stew)

✿ **Rice pilaf** (long-grain rice seasoned with butter and saffron)

✿ **Stewed green beans** (green beans stewed with tomatoes and herbs)

Feta cheese

Kalamata (olives)

✿ **Pita bread**

Desserts

Baklava (pastry made with layers of phyllo dough, nuts, and sugar)

Kataif (pastry made with shredded dough, nuts, and sugar)

Rice pudding

✿ **Turkish coffee**

✿ **American coffee**

················ ◆ **"May I Take Your Order"** ▸ ·················

Low-Calorie Sample Meal

Tabouli
Quantity: ¼ cup
Gyro sandwich with pita bread
Quantity: 3 oz. meat, a 6" pita bread and 2 tbsp. tzatziki sauce

NUTRITION SUMMARY
560 calories
Carbohydrate: 60 g, 42%
Fat: 20 g, 32%
Protein: 36 g, 26%
Cholesterol: 76 mg
Sodium: 1000 mg

Moderate-Calorie Sample Meal

Fattoush (dressing on the side)
Quantity: 1½ cups
Dressing
Quantity: 1 tablespoon
Sheik el Mahshi
Quantity: 1½ cups (½ order)
Kibbeh, baked
Quantity: 1 cup (½ order)
Rice pilaf
Quantity: ⅔ cup
Retsina wine
Quantity: 6 oz.

NUTRITION SUMMARY
830 calories
Carbohydrate: 79 g, 38%
Fat: 30 g, 33%
Protein: 31 g, 15%
Alcohol: 116 (calories), 14%
Cholesterol: 50 mg
Sodium: 1110 mg